Your *Clinics* subs **ter!**

MW01110467

You can now access t **on online at no additional cost! Activate your online subscription today and receive...**

- Full text of all issues from 2002 to the present
- Photographs, tables, illustrations, and references
- Comprehensive search capabilities
- Links to MEDLINE and Elsevier journals

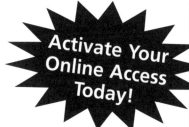

Activate Your Online Access Today!

Plus, you can also sign up for E-alerts of upcoming issues or articles that interest you, and take advantage of exclusive access to bonus features!

To activate your individual online subscription:

1. Visit our website at **www.TheClinics.com**.

2. Click on "Register" at the top of the page, and follow the instructions.

3. To activate your account, you will need your subscriber account number, which you can find on your mailing label (note: the number of digits in your subscriber account number varies from six to ten digits). See the sample below where the subscriber account number has been circled.

This is your subscriber account number

```
************************************3-DIGIT 001
FEB00   J0167   C7   123456-89   10/00   Q: 1

J.H. DOE, MD
531 MAIN ST
CENTER CITY, NY  10001-001
```

4. That's it! Your online access to the most trusted source for clinical reviews is now available.

theclinics.com

ELSEVIER

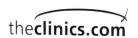

CLINICS IN
PLASTIC SURGERY

Pediatric Plastic Surgery

GUEST EDITORS
Samuel Stal, MD, FACS and
Larry H. Hollier, MD

January 2005 • Volume 32 • Number 1

SAUNDERS

An Imprint of Elsevier, Inc.
PHILADELPHIA   LONDON   TORONTO   MONTREAL   SYDNEY   TOKYO

W.B. SAUNDERS COMPANY
A Division of Elsevier Inc.

The Curtis Center • Independence Square West • Philadelphia, Pennsylvania 19106

http://www.theclinics.com

CLINICS IN PLASTIC SURGERY
January 2005
Editor: Joe Rusko

Volume 32, Number 1
ISSN 0094-1298
ISBN 1-4160-2694-0

Copyright © 2005 Elsevier Inc. All rights reserved. No part of this publication may be reproduced or transmitted in any form or by any means, electronic or mechanical, including photocopy, recording, or any information retrieval system, without written permission from the publisher.

Single photocopies of single articles may be made for personal use as allowed by national copyright laws. Permission of the publisher and payment of a fee is required for all other photocopying, including multiple or systematic copying, copying for advertising or promotional purposes, resale, and all forms of document delivery. Special rates are available for educational institutions that wish to make photocopies for non-profit educational classroom use. Permissions may be sought directly from Elsevier Inc. Rights & Permissions Department, PO Box 800, Oxford OX5 IDX, UK; phone: (+44) 1865 843830, fax: (+44) 1865 853333, e-mail: permissions@elsevier.co.uk. You may also contact Rights & Permissions directly through Elsevier's home page (http://www.elsevier.com), selecting first 'Customer Support', then 'General Information', then 'Persmissions Query Form'. In the USA, users may clear permissions and make payments through the Copyright Clearance Center, Inc., 222 Rosewood Drive, Danvers, MA 01923, USA; phone: (978) 750-8400; fax: (978) 750-4744, and in the UK through the Copyright Licensing Agency Rapid Clearance Service (CLARCS), 90 Tottenham Court Road, London W1P 0LP, UK; phone: (+44) 171 436 5931; fax: (+44) 171 436 3986. Others countries may have a local reprographic rights agency for payments.

Reprints. For copies of 100 or more, of articles in this publication, please contact the Commercial Reprints Department, Elsevier Inc., 360 Park Avenue South, New York, New York 10010-1710. Tel. (212) 633-3813 Fax: (212) 462-1935 email: reprints@elsevier.com

The ideas and opinions expressed in *Clinics in Plastic Surgery* do not necessarily reflect those of the Publisher. The Publisher does not assume any responsibility for any injury and/or damage to persons or property arising out of or related to any use of the material contained in this periodical. The reader is advised to check the appropriate medical literature and the product information currently provided by the manufacturer of each drug to be administered to verify the dosage, the method and duration of administration, or contraindications. It is the responsibility of the treating physician or other health care professional, relying on independent experience and knowledge of the patient, to determine drug dosages and the best treatment for the patient. Mention of any product in this issue should not be construed as endorsement by the contributors, editors, or the Publisher of the product or manufacturers' claims.

Clinics in Plastic Surgery (ISSN 0094-1298) is published quarterly by W.B. Saunders Company. Corporate and editorial offices: The Curtis Center, Independence Square West, Philadelphia, PA 19106-3399. Accounting and circulation offices: 6277 Sea Harbor Drive, Orlando, FL 32887-4800. Periodicals postage paid at Orlando, FL 32862, and additional mailing offices. Subscription prices are $245.00 per year for US individuals, $370.00 per year for US institutions, $123.00 per year for US students and residents, $280.00 per year for Canadian individuals, $420.00 per year for Canadian institutions, $295.00 per year for international individuals, $420.00 per year for international institutions, and $148.00 per year for Canadian and foreign students/residents. To receive student/resident rate, orders must be accompanied by name of affiliated institution, date of term, and the *signature* of program/residency coordinator on institution letterhead. Orders will be billed at individual rate until proof of status is received. Foreign air speed delivery is included in all *Clinics* subscription prices. All prices are subject to change without notice. POSTMASTER: Send address changes to *Clinics in Plastic Surgery*, W.B. Saunders Company, Periodicals Fulfillment, Orlando, FL 32887-4800. **Customer Service: 1-800-654-2452 (US). From outside of the US, call 1-407-345-4000.**

Clinics in Plastic Surgery is covered in *Current Contents, EMBASE/Excerpta Medica, Science Citation Index, Index Medicus, ASCA, and ISI/BIOMED.*

Printed in the United States of America.

GUEST EDITORS

SAMUEL STAL, MD, FACS, Professor, Pediatric Plastic Surgery, Division of Plastic Surgery, Texas Children's Hospital; and Division of Plastic Surgery, DeBakey Department of Surgery, Baylor College of Medicine, Houston, Texas

LARRY H. HOLLIER, MD, Associate Professor, Pediatric Plastic Surgery, Division of Plastic Surgery, Texas Children's Hospital; and Division of Plastic Surgery, DeBakey Department of Surgery, Baylor College of Medicine, Houston, Texas

CONTRIBUTORS

BRUCE S. BAUER, MD, FACS, FAAP, Professor, Department of Surgery, Feinberg School of Medicine, Northwestern University; and Chairman, Division of Plastic Surgery, Children's Memorial Hospital, Chicago, Illinois

RICHARD J. BROWN, MD, Division of Plastic Surgery, Northwestern University School of Medicine; and Department of Surgery, Mount Sinai Hospital, Chicago, Illinois

JAMAL M. BULLOCKS, MD, Brachial Plexus Center, Texas Children's Hospital; and Division of Plastic Surgery, Baylor College of Medicine, Houston, Texas

JULIA CORCORAN, MD, FACS, Assistant Professor, Department of Surgery, Feinberg School of Medicine, Northwestern University; and Attending Surgeon, Division of Plastic Surgery, Children's Memorial Hospital, Chicago, Illinois

GUPREET DHILLON, MD, Brachial Plexus Center, Texas Children's Hospital; and Division of Plastic Surgery, Baylor College of Medicine, Houston, Texas

TUE A. DINH, MD, Assistant Professor, Division of Plastic Surgery, Baylor College of Medicine, Houston, Texas

JEFFREY FRIEDMAN, MD, Assistant Professor, Division of Plastic Surgery, Baylor College of Medicine, Houston, Texas

JAMES T. GOODRICH, MD, PhD, Director, Pediatric Neurologic Surgery, Children's Hospital at Montefiore, Montefiore Medical Center; and Professor, Clinical Neurologic Surgery, Plastic Surgery, and Pediatrics, Albert Einstein College of Medicine, Bronx, New York

ARUN K. GOSAIN, MD, Professor, Department of Plastic Surgery, Medical College of Wisconsin, Milwaukee, Wisconsin

STEPHEN HIGUERA, MD, Research Fellow, Division of Plastic Surgery, Baylor College of Medicine, Houston, Texas

LARRY H. HOLLIER, MD, Associate Professor, Pediatric Plastic Surgery, Division of Plastic Surgery, Texas Children's Hospital; and Division of Plastic Surgery, DeBakey Department of Surgery, Baylor College of Medicine, Houston, Texas

NEIL F. JONES, MD, Chief, Division of Hand Surgery, Department of Orthopedic Surgery, University of California Los Angeles, Los Angeles, California

JOHN Y.S. KIM, MD, Assistant Professor of Surgery, Division of Plastic Surgery, Northwestern University School of Medicine, Chicago, Illinois

JOHN P. LAURENT, MD, Brachial Plexus Center and Chief, Neurosurgery Service, Texas Children's Hospital; and Associate Professor, Department of Pediatric Neurosurgery, Baylor College of Medicine, Houston, Texas

RITA T. LEE, MD, Brachial Plexus Center; and Department of Pediatric Neurology, Texas Children's Hospital, Houston, Texas

KELLY A. LENTON, PhD, Children's Surgical Research Program, Division of Plastic and Reconstructive Surgery, Department of Surgery, Stanford University School of Medicine, Stanford University Medical Center, Stanford, California

JOHN LOGIUDICE, MD, Department of Plastic Surgery, Medical College of Wisconsin, Milwaukee, Wisconsin

MICHAEL T. LONGAKER, MD, MBA, Deane P. and Louise Mitchell Professor and Director, Children's Surgical Research Program, Division of Plastic and Reconstructive Surgery, Department of Surgery, Stanford University School of Medicine, Stanford University Medical Center, Stanford, California

JOSEPH E. LOSEE, MD, FACS, FAAP, Assistant Professor, Departments of Surgery (Plastic) and Pediatrics, University of Pittsburgh; and Chief, Pediatric Plastic Surgery, Children's Hospital of Pittsburgh, Pittsburgh, Pennsylvania

JENNIFER J. MARLER, MD, Division of Plastic Surgery, Department of Surgery, Cincinnati Children's Medical Center, Cincinnati, Ohio

A. CORDE MASON, MD, FAAP, Chief Resident, Division of Plastic Surgery, Department of Surgery, University of Pittsburgh, Pittsburgh, Pennsylvania

JOHN B. MULLIKEN, MD, Professor, Division of Plastic Surgery, Department of Surgery, Children's Hospital and Harvard Medical School, Boston, Massachusetts

RANDALL P. NACAMULI, MD, Children's Surgical Research Program, Division of Plastic and Reconstructive Surgery, Department of Surgery, Stanford University School of Medicine, Stanford University Medical Center, Stanford, California

ROXANA RIVERA, MD, Department of Plastic Surgery, Medical College of Wisconsin, Milwaukee, Wisconsin

A. MICHAEL SADOVE, MD, Professor of Surgery, Division of Plastic Surgery, Indiana University; and Director, Pediatric Plastic Surgery, Indiana University Medical Center, Indianapolis, Indiana

JOSEPH M. SERLETTI, MD, FACS, Professor, Department of Surgery, and Chair, Division of Plastic Surgery, University of Rochester Medical Center, Rochester, New York

SALEH M. SHENAQ, MD, Cofounder and Director, Brachial Plexus Center, Texas Children's Hospital; Professor and Chief, Division of Plastic Surgery; Professor of Neurosurgery; and Professor of Physical Medicine and Rehabilitation, Baylor College of Medicine, Houston, Texas

MELVIN SPIRA, MD, Craniofacial and Cleft Lip and Palate Program, Texas Children's Hospital; and Division of Plastic Surgery, DeBakey Department of Surgery, Baylor College of Medicine, Houston, Texas

DAVID A. STAFFENBERG, MD, Chief, Plastic Surgery and Surgical Director, Center for Craniofacial Disorders, Children's Hospital at Montefiore, Montefiore Medical Center; and Assistant Professor, Plastic Surgery and Pediatrics, Albert Einstein College of Medicine, Bronx, New York

SAMUEL STAL, MD, FACS, Professor, Pediatric Plastic Surgery, Division of Plastic Surgery, Texas Children's Hospital; and Division of Plastic Surgery, DeBakey Department of Surgery, Baylor College of Medicine, Houston, Texas

CONTRIBUTORS

JOHN A. VAN AALST, MD, Assistant Professor of Surgery, Division of Plastic Surgery, University of North Carolina; and Director, Pediatric and Craniofacial Plastic Surgery, University of North Carolina, Chapel Hill, North Carolina

DERRICK C. WAN, MD, Children's Surgical Research Program, Division of Plastic and Reconstructive Surgery, Department of Surgery, Stanford University School of Medicine, Stanford University Medical Center, Stanford, California

ADAM B. WEINFELD, MD, Craniofacial and Cleft Lip and Palate Program, Texas Children's Hospital; and Division of Plastic Surgery, DeBakey Department of Surgery, Baylor College of Medicine, Houston, Texas

CONTENTS

biomedical engineering, tissue engineering, polymer science, molecular biology, developmental biology, and genetics. The goal of this scientific effort is to translate research advances into improved treatments for children with congenital and acquired defects. Although the last decade has seen a dramatic acceleration in research related to pediatric plastic surgery, the next 10 years will no doubt lead to novel treatment strategies with improved clinical outcomes.

FORTHCOMING ISSUES

RECENT ISSUES

THE CLINICS ARE NOW AVAILABLE ONLINE!

Access your subscription at:
www.theclinics.com

ELSEVIER
SAUNDERS

Clin Plastic Surg 32 (2005) xiii

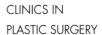
CLINICS IN
PLASTIC SURGERY

Preface

Pediatric Plastic Surgery

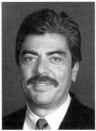 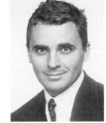

Samuel Stal, MD   Larry H. Hollier, MD
Guest Editors

It is well accepted now that children are not simply little adults. In all aspects, from the psychologic to the physiologic, there are distinct differences that affect their care. With the recognition of this, the treatment of plastic surgical problems in children has developed into a distinct subspecialty. As such, we have chosen a broad range of topics for this issue of the *Clinics in Plastic Surgery*. These topics demonstrate both the unique conditions encountered in children and variations in treatment for those conditions that affect both adults and the pediatric population. The authors have done a magnificent job of bringing together the most current information regarding the management of these reconstructive issues.

Samuel Stal, MD
Professor, Pediatric Plastic Surgery
and
Larry H. Hollier, MD
Associate Professor, Pediatric Plastic Surgery
Division of Plastic Surgery
Texas Children's Hospital
6621 Fannin Street, Suite 620.10
Houston, TX 77030, USA
E-mail addresses: sxstal@texaschildrenshospital.org
(S. Stal)
larryh@bcm.tmc.edu (L.H. Hollier)

0094-1298/05/$ – see front matter © 2005 Elsevier Inc. All rights reserved.
doi:10.1016/j.cps.2004.10.004

ELSEVIER
SAUNDERS

Clin Plastic Surg 32 (2005) 1 – 10

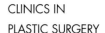
CLINICS IN
PLASTIC SURGERY

Pediatric upper extremity replantation

John Y.S. Kim, MD[a],*, Richard J. Brown, MD[a,b], Neil F. Jones, MD[c]

[a]Division of Plastic Surgery, Northwestern University School of Medicine, 19-250 Galter, 675 North St. Clair Street,
Chicago, IL 60611, USA
[b]Department of Surgery, Mount Sinai Hospital Medical Center, California Avenue at 15th Street, Chicago, IL 60608, USA
[c]Department of Orthopedic Surgery, University of California Los Angeles, 200 UCLA Medical Plaza,
Los Angeles, CA 90024, USA

Reconstruction of complex deformities of the hand has provided a fertile bed for the general evolution of microsurgical technique. Following the pioneering work of Jacobson et al [1], Dongyue et al [2], Buncke et al [3], Komatsu and Tamai [4], Cobbett [5], O'Brien et al [6], and others, the use of microsurgical technique entered the armamentarium of hand surgeons seeking to address both congenital and traumatic deformities of the upper extremity. For traumatic amputation of digits, microvascular replantation has been as fruitful in adults as it has in pediatric patients.

When dealing with microsurgical reconstruction of the pediatric hand vis-à-vis reconstruction of the adult hand, certain anatomic and physiologic issues are pertinent. Although differences in vascular anatomy and physiology exist, there is some controversy as to their real significance in microvascular transfer. Early in the evolution of pediatric microsurgery, Gilbert [7] believed that very small vessels would pose a technical impediment to successful free tissue transfer and advocated a minimum vessel diameter of 0.7 mm, below which he thought that microanastomoses were technically too challenging to be reliably successful. However, large subsequent series have shown that successful flap and digit survival

outcomes can be obtained with smaller vessel calibers. In their series of 106 pediatric microsurgical cases, Canales et al [8] reported that small vessel size (0.2–0.3 mm) led to flap failure in two patients (1.9%). Reversible but presumably problematic vasospasm was reported in another two patients (1.9%). In the authors' experience, the typical size of vessels encountered in most pediatric patients requiring replantation is not a contraindication to microsurgical procedures.

The ease with which vessels in children may undergo vasospasm during microsurgical reconstruction of limbs—both upper and lower—has been well described [9], although other authors have suggested that the relative lack of a muscularis layer may, in fact, minimize vasospasm in pediatric vessels [10,11]. In lower-extremity pediatric microsurgical reconstruction, some surgeons have advocated spinal and locoregional anesthesia, in addition to judicious use of topical lidocaine and papaverine to mitigate vessel irritability—especially in the context of a child in pain, with the presumed concomitant sympathetic discharge (Larry Hollier, MD, personal communication). Rigorous clinical studies addressing this issue have yet to be published.

Indications for pediatric replantation

Although nothing mandates that all extremity amputations in children should be replanted, many

---

* Corresponding author.
E-mail address: jokim@nmh.org (J.Y.S. Kim).

0094-1298/05/$ – see front matter © 2005 Elsevier Inc. All rights reserved.
doi:10.1016/j.cps.2004.09.003

hand surgeons will at least attempt replantation. Early correction of traumatic and congenital deficiencies of the hand may enhance future functional and psycho-social adaptation [12]. However, the same anatomic caveats or restrictions that apply to adults are not applied to children. In adults, there is some question as to the utility of Zone II replantation [13], whereas children are believed to have a greater capacity for healing, which may translate into improved outcomes in marginal replantation situations [14–18]. At the most distal anatomic levels, composite grafting of tip amputations is a viable alternative to the attempted replantation of diminutive vessels [19].

Another parameter that is frequently used to judge candidacy for adult replantation is warm ischemia time. Certainly, warm ischemia predisposes to cel-lular death and reperfusion injury and should there-fore be limited; however, there are anecdotal reports of survival of replanted digits with more than 24 hours of warm ischemia time [20]. This enhanced survival may be due in part to the lack of a muscle component in digital replantation.

Aside from the issue of vessel size, the age of the patient may be a variable worth considering in replantation and pediatric microsurgery in general. Ohmori et al [21] reported performing a free groin flap on a 3-month-old patient, and Lister and Scheker's [22] series of microsurgery for congenital deformities of the hand had a mean patient age of 34 months. No specific age limitation appears to apply to microsurgical intervention, unless it relates to the technical difficulty of vessel size (as described previously). Less clear is the issue of anesthetic complications in the very young. In large series [8,23], no significant morbidity or mortality was associated with microsurgical procedures in the pediatric population.

Technique: replantation of the forearm, hand, and digits

General concepts

Pediatric replantation is predicated on the trau-matic nature of the inciting injury to the extremity; hence, a thorough general trauma evaluation must be made. A review of patients referred to the Buncke Clinic for emergency microsurgery revealed a 1% in-cidence of serious unrecognized injury [24]. Informed discussion and consent are of paramount importance before operative exploration and possible replanta-tion. Often patients are delivered to a microvascular

hand surgeon with the expectation that replantation is the logical extrapolation from transfer for a higher order of care, when, in reality, the decision to replant resides solely with the operating surgeon who as-sesses the feasibility of the reconstruction. The very real potential that replantation may not be possible given the severity of injury (extensive, distal damage to vessels, severe comminution of bone, irreparable nerve damage, loss of joint and tendinous structures) must be communicated to the patient with rigorous informed consent.

Transportation of the amputated part in saline-moistened, cooled gauze is recommended. Judicious use of a pneumatic tourniquet can minimize blood loss: 41% of children undergoing replantation in one series were noted to require postoperative transfu-sions [14]. Before surgery, antibiotic prophylaxis with a first-generation cephalosporin will suffice, and teta-nus prophylaxis should be instituted. Optimally, two teams will be used: one to prepare the amputated segment and the other to explore and ready the re-cipient tissue structures.

Digits

Midlateral incisions allow broad exposure of the digital vessels and nerves. Dorsal veins are found superficially in the subdermal layer of dorsal skin flaps. Bony shortening is important to minimize ten-sion on arteries, veins, and nerves; in children, how-ever, efforts should be made to avoid compromising the epiphyseal plate [13,25–27]. Although miniplates and Kirschner wires can be used to fixate bone, the authors prefer to employ interosseus cerclage wires for stable bony fixation.

Arteries are then addressed. Although sharp lacerations will yield vessel ends suitable for facile anastomosis, the more typical avulsion injuries may lead to significant separation between the proximal and distal ends of the arteries, which may require interposition vein grafts even with the bone short-ening [16,28]. Spare anatomic structures from irrep-arable digits may be a ready source of grafts for both vessels and nerves. The authors prefer to carry out the anastomosis in an interrupted fashion using 10.0 or 11.0 suture, with a single bolus of low-dose heparin given intravenously before anastomotic completion.

The identification and anastomosis of suitable veins is perhaps the most technically demanding part of the replantation, and, in children, these vessels may pose a significant technical obstacle [16,28]. If possible, at least two dorsal veins are anastomosed. In the event that veins cannot be located within the amputated part, proceeding with the arterial anastomosis may stimulate venous engorgement and aid in their location. The importance of venous anastomosis in fingertip replantation, to reduce postoperative congestion and bleeding and thus to improve tip replant survival, is evidenced in a series of 55 patients by Hattori et al [29]. They were able to obtain successful venous repair in 83% of their patients, yielding an overall survival of 86% in fingertip replants [29]. When venous congestion is present or imminent, use of medicinal leeches (*Hirudo medicinalis*) is helpful. Prophylaxis against *Aeromonas hydrophilus* infection should be instituted when leeches are used. Additionally, close monitoring of hemoglobin is required, because prolonged leech therapy can result in significant blood loss.

Tendons may be repaired by means of modified Kessler or another standard technique; if necessary, in the case of avulsed tendons, primary tendon transfer may be performed. It is often useful to repair flexor tendons before extensor tendons. Next in the sequence of repair is coaptation of nerve using 8-0 or 9-0 sutures. If a significant nerve gap exists, immediate nerve grafting is possible with grafts taken from the posterior interosseus nerve or from non-salvageable digits. Other surgeons have reported using the lateral femoral cutaneous nerve, the superficial peroneal nerve on the dorsum of the foot, and the sural nerve with success [30,31]. Otherwise, tagging of the nerves for delayed secondary grafting is an option. In some cases of amputation distal to the distal interphalangeal joint, nerve suturing is not performed because of the anatomic location of the nerve trifurcation. A retrospective analysis in children showed that, even in the absence of nerve suturing, the ability for spontaneous neurotization leading to restoration of sensation and two-point discrimination exists—a finding that strengthens children as candidates for the replantation of distal digits [32]. Skin coverage can be an issue. On rare occasions skin grafts may be required for coverage, but placing them over the vital structures does not generally pose a problem [33]. It is the authors' practice to give aspirin 12 hours after surgery.

Monitoring the digits requires due diligence, with clinical signs such as color, capillary refill, and temperature being crucial to the reliable assessment of survival. Pulse-oximeters or temperature monitors may be used. In the latter case, a temperature below 30°C or a drop of 2° compared with normal digits are hallmarks of digital compromise [34]. Venous outflow is a frequent culprit in digital compromise. In the absence of adequate microvascular salvage of venous drainage, heparin-soaked sponges applied to abraded nailbeds or leech therapy may be necessary to maintain outflow.

Multiple-digit amputations in children can be challenging and frustrating (Fig. 1). The need for special attention to these injuries is accentuated by the loss of function that accompanies them. The goal of multiple-digit replantation should be to restore the hand as close as possible to original function, such as the ability to pinch and grasp [35,36]. That goal mandates that, at the minimum, a thumb and apposing digit be replanted (Fig. 2). Surgeon choice factors into the manner in which multiple-digit replantation is performed. Although structure-by-structure repair of bone, tendon, nerve, and vessel can be performed, the authors favor repair of the thumb followed by repair of the long and ring fingers (and, optionally, of the index and small fingers).

Hand

Hand injuries in children are most commonly of the crush or avulsion type rather than guillotine-type amputations. Once in the operating room, debridement of devitalized tissue should be performed with care to preserve potentially functioning tissue. Pulse lavage may be used at this time to help remove any foreign body or infectious material. The blood supply through the metacarpal region is rich, and replantation at this level should proceed only after hemostasis [37]. In an effort to provide for rapid revascularization, the forearm and one lower extremity should be prepared for potential vein grafting [38]. The focus should then turn toward bone stabilization, which may be extensive and require fixation with Kirschner wires. In cases where amputation occurs at the level of the wrist, reconstruction of long bone may be required. The use of vascularized fibular head and iliac crest grafts has been described [39–42]. Injury to the hand may be so devastating that certain parts will not be replantable. In a review, Epstein et al [43] discuss various uses of spare parts for upper-extremity mutilating injuries. Tissue insult may be so extensive that on healing the hand becomes stiff and dysfunctional, resulting in multiple operations for contracture release and possible toe-to-hand transplantation [44].

Forearm and arm

The technique for replantation of the upper extremity varies slightly from that for the digit or hand. Inducing hypothermia of the replant helps to minimize warm ischemia time; hence many authors advocate submersion in an iced saline solution or cold perfusion with heparinized saline [45,46]. The muscle mass of an amputated extremity, as well as the recipient stump, requires meticulous debridement and timely revascularization with shunting to avoid late revascularization syndrome [47]. The goal of prompt revascularization is to minimize muscle death and the risk of limb infection. Before stabilization, bony ends may need preparation for proper fixation. Again, it is important to avoid epiphyseal plate injury and conseqently to forgo the use of plates and screws at this level [48]. Controversy exists as to whether arterial or venous flow should be restored first. The authors believe that such decisions are best made by surgeons evaluating specific clinical situations. Because limb engorgement is an imminent problem, as many venous anastomoses as possible should be performed, and reverse saphenous grafts should be used judiciously so as not to compromise adequate debridement of vessel ends. Finally, tendons and nerves are sutured; if necessary, sural nerve grafts may be used (Fig. 3) [47–49]. Depending on warm ischemia time, it is almost universal to perform an upper-extremity fasciotomy after tension-free skin

closure, followed by dressing placement and splint immobilization. Anticoagulation medications are not routinely used as with digital replantation. Second-look operations are usually performed several days later to assess the viability of muscle and tissue. In the event that replantation is not possible, prosthetic devices may significantly improve the day-to-day functioning of the patient [50].

Outcomes

Success rates among larger pediatric replantation series range from 63% to 97% (Table 1) [18,47, 51–55]. Favorable prognostic factors for replantation in children under 34 months of age include clean lacerations and body weight greater than 11 kg [14]. This study does not show a correlation between survival and digit position, level of amputation time, or total ischemia time. Ninety percent of the digits that did not survive did so because of avulsion injuries. Cheng et al [18] performed a long-term (average 11 years) functional analysis of digital replantation in children and found that mean total active motion was 130°; 151° for the thumb and fin-

Table 1
Analysis of dedicated pediatric upper-extremity replantation series

Authors	Patients	Mean age or range	Success rate (%)	Functional outcome
Cheng GL et al, 1998	26	4 y	97	Mean total active motion thumb = 120° Mean total active motion fingers = 151° Normal two-point discrimination = 88% Relative grip strength = 79% versus contralateral Activities of daily living = 96% (excellent)
Beris AE et al, 1994	14	2.5 y–16 y	86	Average additional procedures = 2.8
Gary L et al, 1994	33	<34 mo	69	Not available
Saies AD et al, 1994	73	3 d–16 y	63	Average total active motion (including revascularization) = 155° Average two-point discrimination = 8 mm (age-dependent)
Taras JS et al, 1991	120	7 mo–16 y	77	Not available
Wang CQ, 1991	120	Not available	94	Not available
Ikeda et al, 1990	14	4 y	88	Two-point discrimination range = 3–5 mm Tamai classification = 92% (excellent)
Jaeger SH et al, 1981	41	<16 y	85	Average number of additional procedures = 1.0 All with protective sensibility (6/41 with two-point discrimination = 5 mm) Median range total active motion = 90°–180°
O'Brien BM et al, 1980	31	6.8 y	65	Average two-point discrimination = 4 mm Full range of motion = 25% (All data include revascularizations.)

gers. Recovery of sensation to S4 levels was reported in 88% of patients (with two-point discrimination of 4 mm in that cohort). Relative pinch strength versus contralateral controls was 88%; relative grasp strength was 79%. The overall relative length of the replanted digits was 91% of normal when the patients reached maturity.

Saies et al [51] report a large series of 120 children undergoing replantation and revascularization of the upper extremity. As in the Baker study [14], crush/avulsion injuries show a low survival rate (53%) when compared with laceration survival (72%). Replantation and revascularization yielded total average motion of 155° and 172°, respectively, and two-point discrimination averaged 8 mm. The level of injury had no correlation with survival; however, level I injuries (distal to the insertion of the flexor digitorum superficialis) did show superior results compared with level II injuries (distal to the radio-carpal joint, proximal to the flexor digitorum superficialis insertion). In this same study, overall survival of revascularization was superior to replantation survival (88% versus 63%; $P < .0002$).

The prognosis for functional outcome following major replantation is more guarded (Fig. 3). One series showed that a mean of 2.8 additional procedures were needed to improve function following major limb replantation [52]. Moreover, the most common serious complication in this subset patients is the sepsis stemming from myonecrosis—again, the critical anatomic difference in more proximal replantation being the presence of greater muscle mass.

When dealing with the pediatric population, it is important to keep in mind that bones should continue to grow with maturity, if the epiphyseal plate does not close prematurely. Therefore, techniques for osteosynthesis that are used in adults should not always be employed in children. In one series, Chang et al [56] used radiographic analysis to track growth in prior toe-to-hand transplants. They showed that in 96% of transfers epiphyseal plates remained open, and replanted digits grew in concurrence with contralateral controls. A review of the major series involving digital replantation shows that bone-growth rates range from 86% to 93% of contralateral controls [18,54, 55,57]. In a 9-year follow-up study of 12 children undergoing upper-extremity replantation, the longitudinal growth rate of the proximal injured segment was 94.5% of the contralateral side, indicating that skeletal growth can be maintained after replantation [58,59]. However, in a large series of 18 children, 14 of whom had upper-extremity replantation, bone growth was adversely affected when the amputation was complete. Differences in bony growth are mag-

nified at more proximal levels of injury, with one study reporting a 3-cm shortening of bone at 5-year follow-up in patients undergoing forearm replantation [52].

Even when replantation is successful, many complications may occur, leading to secondary operations or loss of the replanted part. When there is compromise of blood flow to tissue, ischemic time increases, and the risk of infection is imminent. The prevailing wisdom is that injuries of the crush/avulsion type cause more damage to tissue than do laceration-type injuries. Several authors report cases of extremity replantation in which limbs were lost because of massive infection from crush injuries [51,52]. Perhaps the most common complications that lead to replantation failure are vascular thrombosis and bleeding [47,54]. Commonly, patients require secondary procedures such as tenolysis for adhesions, tendon grafting, and flap coverage secondary to tissue loss [47,53,54]. Cold intolerance can occur after replantation and has been noted to be as high as 40% in one review [18,54].

Many studies have pointed out that replantation survival is less successful in children than in adults [60,61]. This difference may be due to the nature of injuries in children (crush/avulsion), to their smaller vessels, or even to the aggressive approach we take in deciding whether to perform replantation in children [60,62,63]. Today, microvascular surgery has proved to be a safe procedure in children, with predictable results that allow for one-stage operations and shorter hospital stays. Devaraj et al [10] performed 43 microvascular procedures in 38 children averaging 5.4 years of age and showed an overall vascular success rate of 93%. Hospital stay averaged 10 days and operative time only 5.5 hours.

A single large series of 91 replantations in the upper extremity produced the conclusion that the highest and lowest success rates for replantation are at the levels of the wrist and distal forearm, respectively [17]. Functional outcome of replanted extremities was 80%. Replantation at more proximal levels presents subtly different challenges. On the one hand, the vessels are progressively larger proximally. On the other hand, the presence of muscle in the amputated portion makes the ischemic times much more critical, because muscle begins to undergo significant injury after 6 hours of warm ischemia. Fasciotomies should be part of the armamentarium of proximal replantations [64,65]. In cases where the initial bony fixation and tendon and muscle re-approximation may prolong the ischemic time, arterial inflow may need to be re-established—even with a shunt [65]. The potential

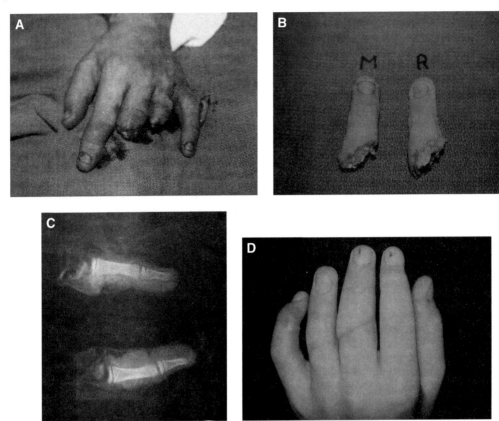

Fig. 1. (*A*) Avulsion amputation of the left middle and ring fingers in an 8 year old girl. (*B*) Amputated left ring and middle fingers. (*C*) Radiograph showing left amputated ring and middle fingers. (*D*) Healed left ring and middle finger replantations.

build-up of toxic metabolites from ongoing muscle ischemia is an indication for performing the arterial anastomoses before venous reconstruction (to prevent the return of these metabolites into the systemic circulation).

Summary

The evolution of microsurgical technique has led to increasing success with pediatric replantation. The broader inclusion criteria for pediatric replanta-

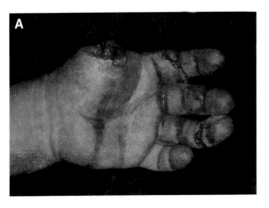

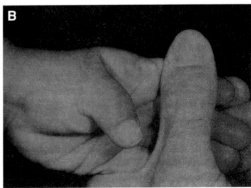

Fig. 2. (*A*) Thumb amputation in a 4 year old boy at the level of the metacarpophalangeal joint. (*B*) Adduction of the replanted thumb.

tion, together with the greater technical demands of repair and the less favorable mechanism of pediatric amputations (crush-avulsion), yield a slightly lower overall survival rate than in adults. The superior nerve and soft tissue regenerative capacity of children appears to produce better functional outcomes. Nonetheless, the issue of cosmesis and developing self-image in a child may have ramifications beyond a simple calculus of range of motion and strength variables—hence the imperative that microsurgical salvage be attempted in pediatric upper-extremity amputations.

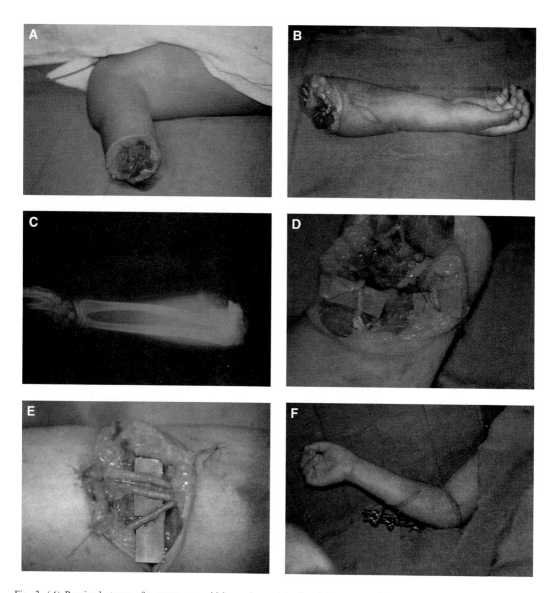

Fig. 3. (A) Proximal stump of a seven year-old boy who sustained a right supracondylar amputation. (B) Amputated limb showing a relatively clean transection at the supracondylar level. (C) Radiograph showing distal humerus transection. (D) Co-aptation of ulnar and radial nerves. (E) Co-aptation of median nerve, anastomoses of brachial artery and two veins. (F) Completed replantation. Note bony fixation secured via an external fixator. (G) Replanted limb at 18 months follow-up. (H) Attempted grasp revealing full finger flexion. (I) Good extension of the fingers at the metacarpophalangeal joints, and limited extension at the interphalangeal joints because the interosseous muscles have not been re-innervated. (J) Full wrist flexion. (K) Full wrist extension. (L) Full elbow flexion. (M) Full elbow extension.

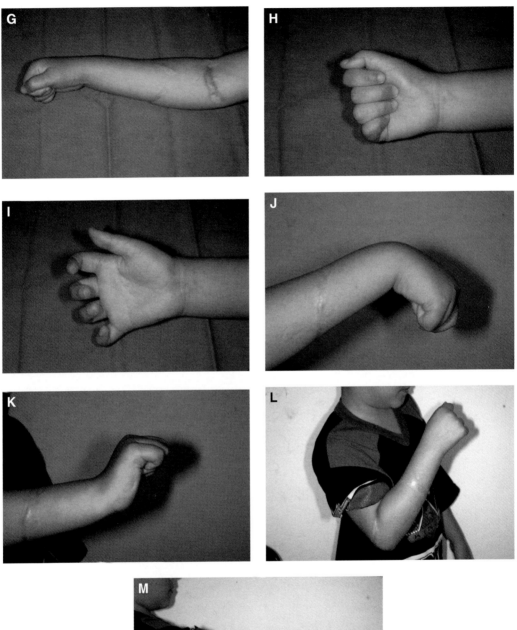

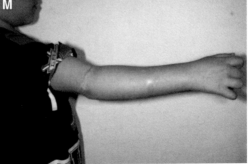

Fig. 3 (*continued*).

References

[1] Jacobson JH, Suarez EL. Results of small artery end-arterectomy-microsurgical technique. Surg Forum 1961;12:256–7.

[2] Dongyue Y, Yudong G. Thumb reconstruction utilizing second toe by microvascular anastomosis: report of 78 cases. Chin Med J [Engl] 1979;92(5):295–309.

[3] Buncke Jr HJ, Schulz WP. Experimental digital amputation and reimplantation. Plast Reconstr Surg 1965; 36:62–70.

[4] Komatsu S, Tamai S. Successful replantation of a completely cut-off thumb. Case report. Plast Reconstr Surg 1968;42:374–7.

[5] Cobbett JR. Free digital transfer. Report of a case of transfer of a great toe to replace an amputated thumb. J Bone Joint Surg 1969;51(B):677–9.

[6] O'Brien BM, Black MJM, Morrison WA, MacLeod AM. Microvascular great toe transfer for congenital absence of the thumb. Hand 1978;10:113–24.

[7] Gilbert A. Reconstruction of congenital hand defects with microvascular toe transfers. Hand Clin 1985;2: 31–60.

[8] Canales F, Lineaweaver C, Furnas H, et al. Microvascular tissue transfer in pediatric patients: analysis of 106 cases. Br J Plast Surg 1991;44:423–7.

[9] Duteille F, Lim A, Dautel G. Free flap coverage of upper and lower limb tissue defects in children: a series of 22 patients. Ann Plast Surg 2003;50:344–9.

[10] Devaraj VS, Kay SP, Batchelor AG, Yates A. Microvascular surgery in children. Br J Plast Surg 1991;44: 276–80.

[11] Parry SW, Toth BA, Elliot LF. Microvascular free tissue transfer in children. Plast Reconstr Surg 1988; 81:838–40.

[12] Boyer MI, Mih AD. Microvascular surgery in the reconstruction of congenital hand anomalies. Hand Clin 1998;14(1):135–42.

[13] Urbaniak JR, Hayes MG, Bright PS. Management of bone in digital replantation: free vascularized and composite bone grafts. Clin Orthop 1978;133:184–94.

[14] Baker GL, Kleinert JM. Digit replantation in infants and young children: determinants of survival. Plast Reconstr Surg 1994;94(1):139–45.

[15] Shenaq SM, Kattash M. Pediatric microsurgery. In: Bentz ML, editor. Pediatric plastic surgery. Stamford (CT): Appleton and Lange; 1998. p. 799–826.

[16] Michalko KB, Bentz ML. Digital replantation in children. Crit Care Med 2002;30(Suppl 11):S444–7.

[17] Wang SH, Young KF, Wei JN. Replantation of severed limbs—clinical analysis of 91 cases. J Hand Surg [Am] 1981;6(4):311–8.

[18] Cheng GL, Pan DD, Zhang NP, Fang GR. Digital replantation in children: a long-term follow-up study. J Hand Surg [Am] 1998;23:635–46.

[19] Heisten JB, Cook PA. Factors affecting composite graft survival in digital tip amputations. Ann Plast Surg 2003;50(3):299–303.

[20] Soucacos PN. Indications and selection for digital amputation and replantation. J Hand Surg [Br] 2001; 26(6):572–81.

[21] Ohmori K, Harii K, Sekigughi J, et al. The youngest free flap yet? Br J Plast Surg 1977;30:273–6.

[22] Lister G, Scheker L. The role of microsurgery in the reconstruction of congenital deformities of the hand. Hand Clinics 1985;1(3):431–42.

[23] Kay SP, Wiberg M. Toe to hand transfer in children. Part 1: Technical aspects. J Hand Surg [Br] 1996;21(6): 723–34.

[24] Partington MT, Lineaweaver WC, O'Hara M, et al. Unrecognized injuries in patients referred for emergency microsurgery. J Trauma 1993;34:238–41.

[25] Tupper JW. Techniques of bone fixation and clinical experience in replanted extremities. Clin Orthop 1978; 133:165–8.

[26] Ikuta Y. Method of bone fixation and re-attachment of amputations in the upper extremities. Clin Orthop 1978;133:169–78.

[27] Meuli HC, Meyer V, Segmuller G. Stabilization of bone in replantation surgery of the upper limb. Clin Orthop 1978;133:179–83.

[28] Cheng GL, Pan DD, Yang ZX, et al. Digital replantation in children. Ann Plast Surg 1985;15(4):325–31.

[29] Hattori Y, Doi K, Ikeda K, et al. Significance of venous anastomosis in fingertip replantation. Plast Reconstr Surg 2003;111(3):1151–8.

[30] Buntic RF, Buncke HJ, Kind GM, et al. The harvest and clinical application of the superficial peroneal sensory nerve for grafting motor and sensory nerve defects. Plast Reconstr Surg 2002;109:145–51.

[31] Yamano Y, Namba Y, Hino Y, et al. Digital nerve grafts in replanted digits. Hand 1982;14(3):255–62.

[32] Faivre S, Lim A, Dautel G, et al. Adjacent and spontaneous neurotization after distal digital replantation in children. Plast Reconstr Surg 2003;111(1):159–65.

[33] Tubiana R. Repair of bilateral hand mutilations. Plast Reconstr Surg 1969;44:323–30.

[34] Lu SY, Chiu HY, Lin TW, Chen MT. Evaluation of survival of digital replantation with thermometric monitoring. J Hand Surg [Am] 1984;9A:805–9.

[35] Bennett JE. Skin and soft tissue injuries of the hand in children. Pediatr Clin North Am 1975;22(2):443–9.

[36] Buncke HJ, Buncke GM, Lineaweaver WC, et al. The contributions of microvascular surgery to emergency hand surgery. World J Surg 1991;15(4):418–28.

[37] Tonkin MA, Ames EL, Wolff TW, Larsen RD. Transmetacarpal amputations and replantation: the importance of the normal vascular anatomy. J Hand Surg [Br] 1988;13B:204–9.

[38] Cooney III WP, Wood MB. Microvascular reconstruction of congenital anomalies and post-traumatic lesions in children. Hand Clin 1992;8(1):131–46.

[39] Gao YH, Ketch LL, Eladoumikdachi F, Netscher DT. Upper limb salvage with microvascular bone transfer for major long-bone segmental tumor resections. Ann Plast Surg 2001;47(3):240–6.

[40] Pederson WC. Upper extremity microsurgery. Plast Reconstr Surg 2001;107(6):1524–37.

[41] Gerwin M, Weiland AJ. Vascularized bone grafts to the upper extremity: indications and technique. Hand Clin 1992;8:509–23.

[42] Tang CH. Reconstruction of the bones and joints of the upper extremity by vascularized free fibular graft: report of 46 cases. J Reconstr Microsurg 1992; 8:285–92.

[43] Epstein W, Chen HC, Chuang CC, Chen HT. Microsurgical reconstruction of distal digits following mutilating hand injuries: results in 121 patients. Br J Plast Surg 1992;3(46):181–6.

[44] Spokevicius S, Radzevicius D. Late toe to hand transfer for the reconstruction of congenital defects of the long fingers. Scand J Plast Reconstr Hand Surg 1997;31(4):345–50.

[45] Rich RH, Knight PJ, Erickson EL, et al. Replantation of the upper extremity in children. J Pediatr Surg 1977; 12(6):1027–32.

[46] Tamai S. Twenty years' experience of limb replantation—review of 293 upper extremity replants. J Hand Surg [Am] 1982;7(6):549–56.

[47] Taras JS, Nunley JA, Urbaniak JR, et al. Replantation in children. Microsurgery 1991;12(3):216–20.

[48] Raimondi PL, Petrolati M, Delaria G. Replantation of large segments in children. Hand Clin 2000;16(4): 547–61.

[49] Daigle JP, Kleinert JM. Major limb replantation in children. Microsurgery 1991;12(3):221–31.

[50] Crandall RC, Tomhave W. Pediatric unilateral below-elbow amputees: retrospective analysis of 34 patients given multiple prosthetic options. J Pediatr Orthop 2002;22(3):380–3.

[51] Saies AD, Urbaniak JR, Nunley JA, et al. Results after replantation and revascularization in the upper extremity in children. J Bone Joint Surg Am 1994;76(12): 1766–76.

[52] Beris AE, Soucacos PN, Malizos KN, et al. Major limb replantation in children. Microsurgery 1994;15(7): 474–8.

[53] Jaeger SH, Tsai TM, Kleinert HE. Upper extremity replantation in children. Orthop Clin North Am 1981; 12(4):897–907.

[54] O'Brien BM, Franklin JD, Morrison WA, MacLeod A. Replantation and revascularization in children. Hand 1980;12(1):12–24.

[55] Ikeda K, Yamauchi S, Hashimoto F, et al. Digital replantation in children: a long-term follow-up study. Microsurgery 1990;11(4):261–4.

[56] Chang J, Jones NF. Radiographic analysis of growth in pediatric microsurgical toe-to-hand transfers. Plast Reconstr Surg 2002;109(2):576–82.

[57] Nunley JA, Spiegl PV, Goldner RD, Urbaniak JR. Longitudinal epiphyseal growth after replantation and transplantation in children. J Hand Surg [Am] 1987; 12(2):274–9.

[58] Demiri E, Bakhach J, Tsakoniatis N, et al. Bone growth after replantation in children. J Reconstr Microsurg 1995;11(2):113–22.

[59] Nagase T, Sekiguchi J, Ohmori K. Finger replantation in a 12-month-old child: a long-term follow-up. Br J Plast Surg 1996;49(8):555–8.

[60] Urbaniak JR. Replantation in children. In: Serafin D, Georgiade N, editors. Pediatric plastic surgery. St. Louis (MO): CV Mosby; 1984. p. 1168–85.

[61] Weiland AJ, Villareal-Rios A, Kleinert HE, et al. Replantation of digits and hand. Analysis of surgical techniques and functional results in 71 patients with 86 replantations. J Hand Surg [Am] 1978;2:1–12.

[62] Gaul J, Pan D, Yang Z, et al. Digital replantation in children. Ann Plast Surg 1985;15:325–31.

[63] Tamai S, Hon Y, Tasumi Y, et al. Microvascular anastomosis and its application on the replantation of amputated digits and hand. Clin Orthop 1978;133: 106–21.

[64] Wood M. Finger and hand replantation: surgical technique. Hand Clin 1992;8(3):397–408.

[65] Goldner RD, Nunley JA. Replantation proximal to the wrist. Hand Clin 1992;8(3):413–25.

ELSEVIER
SAUNDERS

Clin Plastic Surg 32 (2005) 11 – 18

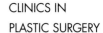

CLINICS IN
PLASTIC SURGERY

Treatment of large and giant nevi

Bruce S. Bauer, MD, FACS, FAAP[a,b,*], Julia Corcoran, MD, FACS[a,b]

[a]Feinberg School of Medicine at Northwestern University, Chicago, IL, USA
[b]Division of Plastic Surgery, The Children's Memorial Hospital, 2300 Children's Plaza, Chicago, IL 60614, USA

Congenital melanocytic nevi (CMN) are composed of clusters of nevo-melanocytes that are generally present at birth but occasionally arise as late as several years. These lesions arise from melanocytic stem cells that migrate from the neural crest to the embryonic dermis and upward into the epidermis [1]. They may also migrate into the leptomeninges. Although small pigmented nevi are present in 1 in 100 births [2], large nevi are present in only 1 in 20,000 births [3], and the giant lesions are even less common [4]. As a result, most surgeons have little experience with them and little opportunity to develop a rational protocol for their treatments.

The appearance of these dark, often hairy lesions over a large portion of a newborn infant's face, trunk, or extremity is often devastating to parents who have been anxiously awaiting the birth of their child. Early consultation with a pediatric plastic surgeon or pediatric dermatologist can help educate the family and decrease the stress of the situation by providing concise information about the nature of the nevus, its natural history, and the options for its management. Families can accept even the news of a multiple-stage reconstruction over many years if it is presented in a compassionate manner.

In nearly 25 years of pediatric plastic surgery practice, the senior author has had the opportunity to treat over 270 children with large and giant pigmented nevi. This experience has afforded the opportunity to compare various treatment approaches and determine which techniques have been most effective in achieving optimal aesthetic and functional outcomes. This article discusses the rationale for treatment and summarizes the authors' current thoughts on planning and accomplishing their treatment goals.

Definitions of size

It is important to have a frame of reference in discussing the treatment of CMN. Multiple definitions have been used, and without some uniformity it is difficult to compare different studies. The authors believe that the following definitions are becoming accepted and used in most studies: Small nevi are those measuring 1.5 cm or less, medium nevi measure from 1.5 to 19.9 cm, and large nevi are 20 cm or greater [5]. Giant nevi are a subset of large nevi that measure 50 cm or greater [4]. Another definition of large and giant nevi classifies them as those that cover 2% or more of total body surface [3,6,7].

During the first 6 months of life, some nevi can appear to "grow" significantly as tardive pigment becomes more visible. Some satellite nevi may become visible for the first time over the first 2 to 3 years (tardive CMN) [4]. After the first 6 months, the lesions grow proportionally to the particular area of the body involved. The diameter of the lesion grows by a factor of 1.7 times in the head, 3.3 in the thigh and leg, and 2.8 in the torso, arms, hands, and feet. The large nevi are at least 6 cm in diameter on the infant's body and 9 cm on its head [4].

* Corresponding author. Division of Plastic Surgery, Children's Memorial Hospital, 2300 Children's Plaza, Box 93, Chicago, IL 60614.
  E-mail address: bbauer@northwestern.edu (B.S. Bauer).

0094-1298/05/$ – see front matter © 2005 Elsevier Inc. All rights reserved.
doi:10.1016/j.cps.2004.08.004

Rationale for and timing of treatment

Two immediate concerns face the family of a child with a large or giant nevus. The first is the risk of the child's developing melanoma [3–9], and the second is the stigma of this very visible lesion and how it will affect the child's psychological development. Although the exact risk of malignant melanoma may never be determined, the early treatment of these lesions, provided it leads to the necessary aesthetic and functional outcome, may alleviate concerns about the child's appearance and significantly reduce the risk of malignant degeneration [6,7,10].

In the literature, the estimated risk of developing melanoma ranges from 2% to 31% [3–7]. The different populations and numbers in these studies explain the wide variance. In a retrospective study, Quaba and Wallace [3] examined patients with CMN covering more than 2% of the total body surface and found the melanoma risk to be 8.5% during the first 15 years of life. Sandsmark et al [11] have quoted a risk of 6.7% in childhood. Marghoob et al [4] have quoted a lifetime risk of 4.5% to 9% for melanoma arising in large and giant CMN. Approximately 50% of the malignancies that develop in large CMN do so in the first 3 years of life [12], 60% by childhood, and 70% by puberty [12,13].

Another factor that needs to be considered and discussed with families is the issue of neurocutaneous melanosis (NCM). Recent reports have demonstrated the association of nevus cells in the leptomeninges in a percentage of children with large nevi in an axial orientation or those with an extensive number of satellite nevi [14–16]. Although symptomatic NCM is characterized by mental retardation, hydrocephalus, and seizures, many children are asymptomatic [14,15]. These children can be identified by T_1 shortening in MR imaging. Foster et al [15] reported that 23% of at-risk patients had evidence of central nervous system involvement (melanotic rests within the brain and meninges) on MR imaging. Marghoob and Dusza [17] have seen this finding in only 3% of children in the Nevus Outreach Registry of over 600 patients. The latter figure coincides with the authors' experience. Although the presence of a lesion on MRI does not typically alter the decision to treat or not treat a child with a large or giant nevus, the approach may be altered in cases of symptomatic NCM.

The rationale for early treatment of large and giant nevi has four components. These are (1) the presence of the greatest risk for malignancy in the first 3 years, (2) the elasticity and healing capacity of the skin in the early years, (3) the greater patient tolerance of surgery at this time, and (4) the psychological benefit [6,7]. Taking all this into account, and assuming the child is otherwise healthy, the authors begin treatment of the large and giant nevus by 6 months of age in most cases, provided they have seen the child from early infancy. Although many of the tissue-expansion procedures used in treatment of giant nevi can be applied to older children and selected adults, the intolerance for repeated procedures and the decreased elasticity of the skin may make the excision of extensive lesions impractical in older patients.

Treatment of large and giant nevi

The treatment of large and giant nevi is controversial [3–12]. Many feel that the risk of degeneration is too low to warrant the unsightly scars or grafts that may follow treatment. Others feel that, in the presence of NCM, the greatest risk lies within the central nervous system, so the excision of the cutaneous lesion can only have limited benefits. However, the appearance of these lesions clearly produces a stigma with significant psychological implications. Removal on this basis is often warranted. The challenge for the surgeon involved in treating these often complex lesions is to develop treatment modalities that not only accomplish the excision of all or most of the nevus but also lead to an optimal aesthetic and functional outcome. Where the second requirement cannot readily be met, it is best not to operate and to have the child closely followed by a dermatologist with experience with giant nevi.

Treatment choices include observation, dermabrasion [18] or curettage [19], and staged excision and reconstruction [6,7,10,12]. Some giant nevi are so extensive as to have no available normal "donor" tissue for reconstruction. In other cases, the family situation or lack of available resources may speak for a less "aggressive" approach. The treating physician should be well versed in the available treatment options, honest about the potential risks and outcomes of the various surgical modalities of treatment, and able to present these to the family or patient (when the latter is old enough to understand).

Dermabrasion [18] and curettage [19] are both techniques that have been applied in the neonatal period in an effort to remove the more concentrated population of nevus cells near the lesion's surface. The technique can be effective in reducing the overall nevus "cell load" but cannot fully remove the nevus, because of the well-known depth of nevus cells in CMN [20]. Although this treatment may result in significant lightening of the color of the lesion, it is quite common to see later "bleed-through" of the deeper nevus, with gradual darkening and reappearance of the lesion. This result may present a difficult treatment problem in visible areas like the face, where other techniques for excision may then be less well tolerated.

Many large and giant nevi can be excised completely or nearly completely with very acceptable aesthetic outcomes. In 1988, the authors presented an overview of their first 78 patients with large and giant nevi (2% of total body surface or greater), focusing on the issue of which treatment techniques most effectively allowed early excision and reconstruction [6]. Since that time, the senior author has treated an additional 193 patients, for a total of 271 patients, and during the intervening 16 years he has modified the treatment approach to address the challenge mentioned earlier. The optimal choice of treatment still varies by body region, and the remainder of this article summarizes the authors' thoughts on these different treatment modalities.

Scalp

Tissue expansion is well recognized as the treatment modality of choice for excision and reconstruction of large and giant nevi of the scalp. As surgical experience increases and planning improves, larger nevi can be excised and the defects reconstructed with fewer serial excisions and better restoration of normal hair patterns. Rectangular expanders with remote injection ports are used here and in all other body regions, with the expanders in place for an average of 10 weeks. Expanders are typically injected weekly (increased to every 4 to 5 days in some cases). The typical expanders used in the scalp vary from 250 to 500 mL in size. Treatment starts as early as 6 months, with some cranial molding expected by the time the expanders are removed, but with no instance of long-term cranial deformity noted (remodeling usually occurs over 3 to 4 months). The most significant modification the authors have made in their technique from early cases to the present is the increased use of expanded transposition flaps rather than advancement flaps [21]. The benefit of this modification is most apparent in the use of the expanded occipital transposition flap for coverage of the entire parietal scalp and reconstruction of the temporal hairline and sideburn. Although it

is not always possible following a single expansion, this approach has been successful in multiple cases and provides for an optimal hair direction and hairline.

Face

Large and giant nevi of the face present some of the greatest challenges in treatment of these lesions. Certainly, these are the most visible nevi with which the patient and family must deal and the ones that are most likely to be associated with significant psychological sequelae. They also represent the area where unsightly scarring is most readily visible; consequently, the planning and execution of the reconstructive plan must be very detailed. A description of all the nuances of treatment of facial nevi is beyond the scope of this paper; this topic has been covered previously in both the authors' work [10] and that of Zuker et al [22]. What follows is a summary of the highlights.

Tissue expansion of the hemiforehead for unilateral lesions or the bilateral or lateral forehead for central lesions can very effectively treat even extensive lesions. Because many of these nevi involve the adjacent scalp, the combined "attack" on both of these regions often facilitates the excision and lessens the number of stages required. Flap advancement, rotation, and transposition each play a role in assuring that the hairline, eyebrow, and distance between the two are not disturbed. Nevi of the cheek are best reconstructed with expanded or nonexpanded postauricular/neck flaps. The reconstruction of the entire aesthetic unit of the cheek may require two expansions. Again, the use of a transposition flap significantly reduces the risk of downward traction and distortion of the lower eyelid and canthus, which are seen as common sequelae of direct advancement of expanded flaps from below the mandible to the cheek.

Expanded or unexpanded full-thickness skin grafts [23] have been used effectively for excision and reconstruction of nevi of the periorbital and eyelid area and, occasionally, of the nasal dorsum. Although single lids may be grafted from a postauricular donor site, a single large expanded full-thickness graft from the supraclavicular area can reconstruct eyelids, canthus, and the region between eyelid and brow without the multiple "seams" that follow the use of many smaller grafts. Recently, the authors have combined the excision of nevi of the lateral forehead and nasal dorsum, borrowing part of the expanded forehead flap to cover the nasal dorsum while advancing the remainder to the temporal area.

Extensive nevi of the central face (nose, lips, chin) are some of the most challenging that we have to deal with, and their treatment requires both ingenuity and a solid grasp of plastic surgery reconstructive techniques.

Trunk

As the authors' series of cases enlarged and their opportunities to view the long-term outcomes of earlier cases increased, it became clear that the role of skin grafting has significantly decreased [7,21]. Physicians need to decide whether the aesthetic and functional outcome of a trunk covered with split-thickness grafts (or, even worse, with meshed split-thickness grafts) is an acceptable alternative to leaving the nevus untreated. If one follows the authors' earlier approach of using large segments of nonmeshed split-thickness skin and confines its use to the back, then the aesthetic outcome may be acceptable. However, the authors confine use of this treatment to cases that are so extensive in size as to have no expandable skin available, and where particularly atypical features of the nevus prompt resection. Today, these cases are few and far between.

Tissue expansion can be very effective on the anterior trunk, provided that the lesion is confined either to the lower abdomen or central abdomen and that there is sufficient uninvolved skin above or above and below the nevus to expand. Expansion must be avoided in or around the area of the breast bud in females, and lesions of the breast should be left until after breast development, regardless of the psychological implications of delaying the treatment till that age.

The use of expanded transposition flaps has allowed excision of nevi of the upper back and buttock/perineal region, where previously it was thought that only skin grafting was possible [21]. Tissue expanders in the 500- to 750-mL range are used most commonly in infants and young children. Serial expansion with careful planning has made possible the excision of progressively larger nevi of the back and buttocks, with excellent outcomes. Another tool for reconstruction of giant nevi of the upper back, shoulders, and neck has been the expanded free transverse rectus abdominus myocutaneous (TRAM) flap, which can be positioned in the upper back and posterior neck or shoulder, then re-expanded, contoured, and draped about the neck and shoulders [24].

Extremities

Large and giant nevi of the extremities present a challenge that is still not fully met. In past years, the authors were willing to excise extensive circumferential nevi of the extremities (both upper and lower) and replace the nevus with either nonmeshed split-thickness skin grafts or large expanded full-thickness skin grafts. However, long-term follow-up of these patients typically demonstrated contour deformities and unacceptable aesthetic outcomes. Concerns were also expressed about both the durability of these grafts and their ability to keep up with normal extremity growth.

Tissue expansion has been of some help in treatment of smaller lesions, where there is available tissue proximal and distal to the lesion and the lesion is confined to a fairly small segment of the limb. The geometry of the extremity, as well as the limited flexibility of the skin (particularly in the lower extremity) makes regional expansion of limited use [24].

In the past decade, the authors have begun to find a way around these limitations, using large expanded transposition flaps from the scapular region to cover the upper arm and shoulder and expanded or non-expanded pedicle flaps from the flank and abdomen for circumferential nevi from the elbow to the wrist. Expanded full-thickness skin grafts have been used effectively for the dorsum of the hand, with excellent aesthetic outcomes [23,24].

Although pedicled flaps are not readily available for coverage of more extensive lesions of the arm, thigh, or leg, the authors have had some success with expanded free flaps from the abdomen and scapular region [24]. These procedures have been used only in very carefully selected cases, and the optimum timing of these complex reconstructive procedures is still under consideration. Again, we must critically evaluate each case and be assured that the treatment chosen is likely to provide an aesthetic and functional outcome that is better than accepting the lesion and dealing with the associated psychological issues with appropriate support.

Satellite nevi

Satellite nevi may appear anywhere over the course of the first few years of life, and their number seems to correlate directly with the likelihood of NCM [16]. They may vary in size from small to medium lesions. To date, no case of melanoma has been reported arising in a satellite nevus [16,17]. With this in mind, it is generally agreed that the primary reason for excision is an aesthetic one. The authors generally excise some of the larger lesions early, often with serial excision, and leave the smaller lesions until the child expresses specific concerns about them. A significant benefit may also result from excising multiple satellite nevi on the face before the child enters his or her school years.

Summary

Although the exact risk of malignant degeneration may never be determined, there is still evidence that large and giant nevi carry this potential. Excision and reconstruction are warranted, provided that they can be accomplished with an optimal aesthetic and functional outcome, but experience has demonstrated that some extensive lesions are best left to observation by the dermatologist (with selective surgery if atypical areas arise). NCM is a well-recognized disorder whose full implications have yet to be determined, but children with large and giant nevi, particularly in axial distribution, should be evaluated. The same goes for those with multiple satellite nevi. The presence of NCM is not at present a contraindication to treating the cutaneous lesion.

Experience with a large population of children with large and giant CMN has demonstrated that thoughtful application of the full spectrum of reconstructive options, heavily weighted toward the use of tissue expansion (as well as expanded pedicled and free flaps) can result in total or near-total excision of many of these extensive nevi with predictably good outcomes (Figs. 1–4).

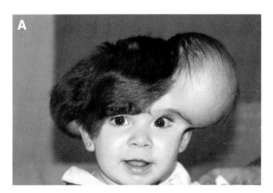
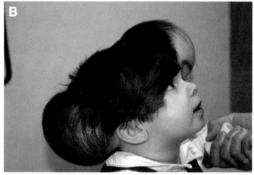
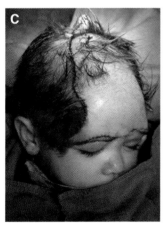
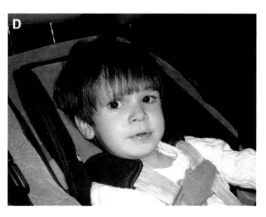

Fig. 1. (*A,B*) One-year-old child with giant nevus of forehead and scalp, with two expanders in place for first-stage excision of nevus following 12 weeks of expansion. (*C*) The expanded forehead flap and scalp flaps in position following excision of the greater part of the nevus. The remaining nevus is in the right lateral forehead and temporal region. (*D*) Appearance 9 months after excision of remaining nevus, with symmetric hairline and brow position.

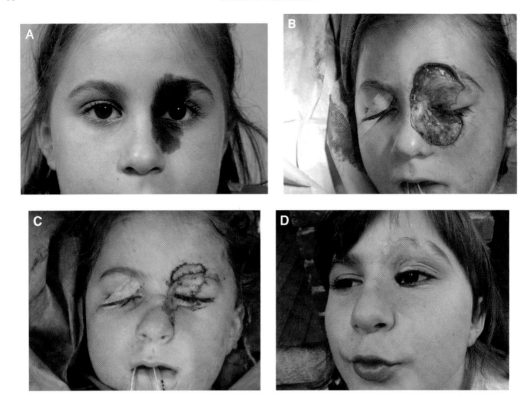

Fig. 2. (*A*) Six-year-old child with large nevus of left medial eyelids and brow, with extension to canthus and lateral nose. (*B*) Defect following excision of the nevus. (*C*) Reconstruction with single large postauricular full-thickness skin graft (FTSG; donor site closed with additional FTSG from groin). Medial brow reconstructed with island flap from temporal region. (*D*) Eight months after the reconstruction, the full-thickness graft is blending in well and has fully reconstructed the complex contours of the defect and lids. The hair growth in the reconstructed brow is still sparse but appears to be increasing. As typically planned in these cases, the nevus of the ciliary margin is left in place to avoid potential functional disturbance of the lid and canalicular function.

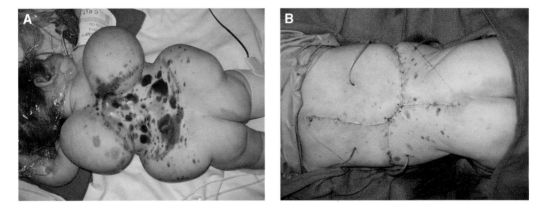

Fig. 3. (*A*) A giant nevus of the back with atypical and variegated pigmentation is approached with placement of four expanders (2–500 mL above and 2–350 mL distal to the nevus). (*B*) The greater part of the nevus is excised following this first expansion, which was carried out over 12 weeks. The remaining nevus will be excised with a second round of expanders after 4 to 6 months of healing.

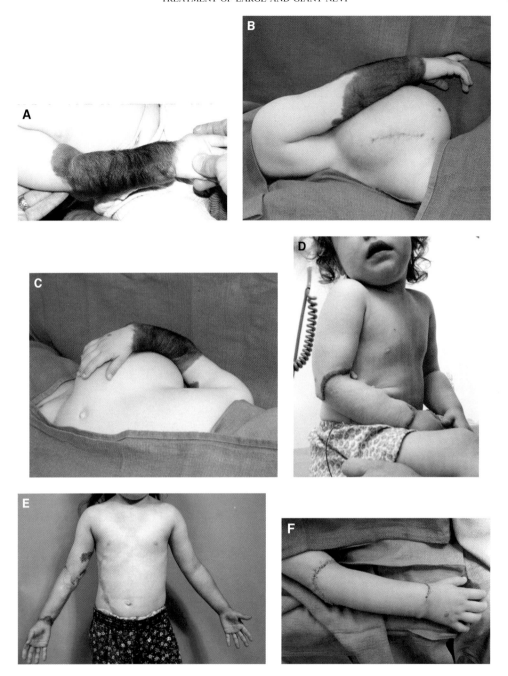

Fig. 4. (*A*) A 2-and-a-half-year-old with a giant nevus extending circumferentially around the forearm from elbow to wrist, with additional satellite nevus in the upper arm. (*B,C*) The arm is positioned against the flank and abdomen after expansion of the site and before placement of the arm within the expanded pedicle flap. (*D*) The arm is placed for 3 weeks within the expanded "tunnel," and the pedicle is gradually tightened with through-and-through bolster sutures, gradually reducing the blood flow through the pedicle. (*E*) The volar surface of the reconstructed forearm with the healing donor site visible on the abdomen. Residual nevus is still present at the wrist and elbow and at the satellite. (*F*) The remaining border of nevus at the edges of the flap is excised. Clearly noted are the excellent contour and quality of the skin of the forearm gained with this approach.

References

[1] Cramer SF. Speckled lentiginous nevus (Nevus spilus): the "roots of the melanocytic garden." Arch Dermatol 2001;137:1654–5.

[2] Castilla EE, Dutra MDG, Orioli-Parreiras ID. Epidemiology of congenital pigmented naevi. I. Incidence rates and relative frequencies. Br J Dermatol 1981; 104:307–15.

[3] Quaba AA, Wallace AF. The incidence of malignant melanoma (0–15 years of age) arising in "large" congenital nevocellular nevi. Plast Reconstr Surg 1986;78:174–9.

[4] Marghoob AA, Kopf AW, Bittencourt FV. Moles present at birth: their medical significance. Skin Cancer Foundation J 1999;36:95–8.

[5] Kopf AW, Bart RS, Hennessey P. Congenital nevocytic nevi and malignant melanomas. J Am Acad Dermatol 1979;1:123–30.

[6] Bauer BS, Vicari FA. An approach to excision of congenital giant pigmented nevi in infancy and early childhood. Plast Reconstr Surg 1988;82:1012–21.

[7] Bauer BS, Byun MY, Han H, Vicari FA. A new look into the treatment of congenital giant pigmented nevi in infancy and childhood: a follow-up study and review of 200 patients. Plast Surg Forum 1997;20:76.

[8] Watt AJ, Kotsis SV, Chung KC. Risk of melanoma arising in large melanocytic nevi: a systematic review. Plast Reconstr Surg 2004;113:1968–74.

[9] Marghoob AA, Schoenbach SP, Kopf AW, et al. Large congenital melanocytic nevi and the risk for the development of malignant melanoma: a prospective study. Arch Dermatol 1996;132:170–5.

[10] Bauer BS, Few JW, Chavez CD, Galiano RD. The role of tissue expansion in the management of large congenital pigmented nevi of the forehead in the pediatric patient. Plast Reconstr Surg 2001;107:668–75.

[11] Sandsmark M, Eskeland G, Ogaard AR, et al. Treatment of large congenital naevi. Scand J Plast Reconstr Hand Surg 1993;27:223–32.

[12] Kaplan EN. The risk of malignancy in large congenital nevi. Plast Reconstr Surg 1974;53:421–8.

[13] Trozak DJ, Rowland WR, Hu F. Metastatic malignant melanoma in prepubertal children. Pediatrics 1975;55: 191–204.

[14] Kadonaga JN, Frieden IJ. Neurocutaneous melanosis: definition and review of the literature. J Am Acad Dermatol 1991;24:747–55.

[15] Foster RD, Williams ML, Barkovich AJ, et al. Giant congenital melanocytic nevi: the significance of neurocutaneous melanosis in neurologically asymptomatic children. Plast Reconstr Surg 2001;107:933–41.

[16] Marghoob AA, Dusza SW, Oliveria SO, Halpern AC. Number of satellite nevi as a correlate for neurocutaneous melanocytosis in patients with large congenital melanocytic nevi. Arch Derm 2004;140: 171–5.

[17] Dusza SW, Marghoob AA. The epidemiology of LCMN. Presented at Nevus Outreach, Inc. meeting. Columbus (OH), July 2004.

[18] Johnson HA. Permanent removal of pigmentation from giant naevi by dermabrasion in early life. Br J Plast Surg 1977;30:321–3.

[19] Casanova D, Bardot J, Andrac-Meyer L, Magalon G. Early curettage of giant congenital naevi in children. Br J Dermatol 1998;138:341–5.

[20] Rhodes AR, Wood WC, Sober AJ, Mibry Jr MC. Nonepidermal origin of malignant melanoma associated with giant congenital nevocellular nevus. Plast Reconstr Surg 1981;67:782–90.

[21] Bauer BS, Margulis A. The expanded transposition flap: shifting paradigms based on experience gained from two decades of pediatric tissue expansion. Plast Reconstr Surg 2004;114:98–106.

[22] Zuker RM, Iconomou TG, Michelow B. Giant congenital pigmented nevi of the face: operative management and risk of malignancy. J Canadien De Chirurgie Plast 1995;3:39–44.

[23] Bauer BS, Vicari FA, Richard ME. Expanded full-thickness skin grafts in children: case selection, planning, and management. Plast Reconstr Surg 1993; 92:59–69.

[24] Margulis A, Bauer BS, Fine NA. Large and giant congenital pigmented nevi of the upper extremity: an algorithm to surgical management. Ann Plast Surg 2004;52:158–67.

ELSEVIER
SAUNDERS

CLINICS IN
PLASTIC SURGERY

Clin Plastic Surg 32 (2005) 19 – 23

International trends in the treatment of cleft lip and palate

Adam B. Weinfeld, MD[a,b], Larry H. Hollier, MD, FACS[a,b],
Melvin Spira, MD[a,b], Samuel Stal, MD, FACS[a,b],*

[a]Craniofacial and Cleft Lip and Palate Program, Texas Children's Hospital, 6621 Fannin Street, Houston, TX 77030, USA
[b]Division of Plastic Surgery, DeBakey Department of Surgery, Baylor College of Medicine, Houston, TX 77030, USA

Of all the procedures that fall under the umbrella of plastic surgery, the goal of restoration of form as well as function is perhaps most germane to cleft lip and palate surgery. Satisfactory results depend on cleft type, the technique used for repair, the experience of the surgeon, and the timing of the repair. Extensive knowledge of the pathologic and normal nasal and oral anatomy, scar formation, and facial development is mandatory. Despite the long history of cleft surgery and the significant psychosocial and aesthetic impact of cleft repair, no standard protocols for surgical management of the cleft patient exist. Recently, surveys evaluating the type of care delivered to cleft patients have been published. These serve as enlightening views on the contemporary state of the art of cleft lip and palate surgery. This article presents the results of an international survey created to evaluate trends in cleft surgery. It compares the data with those of a similar survey by the senior author that was published 6 years ago and with a more recent study evaluating the European cleft experience, in an attempt to identify trends in cleft care [1,2].

International trends

Survey

To gauge international trends in cleft lip and palate surgery, a one-page anonymous survey was mailed to 224 cleft centers in the United States and 34 international cleft centers recognized by the Cleft Lip and Palate Society. All studies were completed in the year 2004. The questions focused primarily on surgical timing and techniques used. The survey response rate was 54.5% (Table 1). Collectively, the centers represented in the survey account for the care of 6432 new patients each year. The survey revealed both considerable variety and several areas of significant consensus with regard to timing and technique in various aspects of cleft care. These differences and similarities in treatment are illustrated in the category-specific survey discussion that follows.

Preoperative orthopedic appliances

Fifty-seven percent of the centers routinely use presurgical appliances (Table 2). Many centers reported using only the passive nasoalveolar molding (NAM) or active Latham-type appliances [3,4]. NAM is employed by 60.8% of the surgeons, and the Latham type of active appliance is used by 24.3% of the surgeons. Eight percent of the centers employed passive and active appliances in their practice, but not necessarily in the same patient.

* Corresponding author. Clinical Care Center, Suite 620, 6621 Fannin Street, MC-CC620.10, Houston, TX 77030.
   E-mail address: sxstal@texaschildrenshospital.org (S. Stal).

0094-1298/05/$ – see front matter © 2005 Elsevier Inc. All rights reserved.
doi:10.1016/j.cps.2004.08.002

Table 1
Survey statistics

Survey response rate	54.6%
Number of centers represented	141
New patients treated each year	6432

Lip adhesion

Although a significant number of centers (43%) report the use of lip adhesion in their practice (Table 3), the total number of patients treated with this modality is probably low; 74% of those who use lip adhesion reported using it in fewer than 10% of their patients. The use of presurgical appliances in the center did not translate into an absence of lip adhesion in the treatment armamentarium. Many centers that used appliances also performed lip adhesion for select cases. The most common reasons for performing lip adhesion include the presence of a wide cleft (48.2%), poor compliance with an appliance or lack of appliance availability (14.3% and 7.1%, respectively), and presence of a bilateral cleft or a bilateral cleft with a prominent premaxilla (10.7% each).

Unilateral cleft lip

In the care of patients with unilateral cleft lips, 33.3% of the centers perform the definitive lip procedure before 3 months of age, 65.9% between 3 and 6 months, and 0.7% at an age greater than 6 months (Table 4). The majority of the centers (84.2%) rely on the Millard rotation-advancement method or some modification of it for lip repair [5,6]. The remaining 14.4% of the surgeons report using the triangular flap or straight-line techniques for primary repair of unilateral cleft lips.

Bilateral cleft lip

The age distribution for the repair of bilateral cleft lips is similar to that for unilateral cleft lip repair.

Table 2
Presurgical orthopedics

Centers using presurgical appliance (%)	57.4
NAM (%)	60.8
Latham (%)	24.3
NAM and/or Latham (%)	8.1
Nonspecified (%)	6.7

Table 3
Lip adhesion

Centers employing lip adhesion (%)	43.3
Indication for lip adhesion (%)	
Wide cleft	48.2
Poor compliance with appliance	14.3
Prominent premaxilla	10.7
Bilateral cleft	10.7
No appliance available	7.1
Other	8.9
Patients per center with lip adhesion (%)	
<10 %	74
11–80 %	14
81–100 %	12

Only 23.1% of the centers perform the closure on patients less than 3 months of age (Table 5). Seventy-six percent of the centers perform the lip repair between 3 and 6 months, and a nominal number undertake repair after 6 months of life. The most frequent method of repair is the rotation advancement (72%) [7]. Triangular flap or straight-line repair was performed as a primary procedure in 28% of the programs.

Cleft nose

The lower lateral cartilage is repositioned at the time of the initial lip repair in 88.3% of the centers (Table 6). When the lower lateral cartilage is not repaired at the same time as the definitive lip repair, the most frequent ages reported for repositioning were 4 years (45.4%) and 5 years (27.3%). Very few centers waited beyond 6 years for alar repositioning (9%). The surgeons were asked for their opinion regarding the age of septal maturity in cleft patients [8]. The average male age reported was 14.4 years (range = 7–20 years), and the average female age reported was 13.4 years (range = 7–19 years).

Table 4
Unilateral cleft lip management

Age of definitive repair (%)	
<3 mo	33.3
3–6 mo	65.9
>6 mo	0.7
Technique (%)	
Rotation advancement	84.2
Straight line/Triangle flap	15.4

Table 5
Bilateral cleft lip management

Age of definitive repair (%)	
<3 mo	23.1
3–6 mo	76.1
>6 mo	0.7
Technique (%)	
Rotation advancement	72
Straight line/Triangle flap	28

Cleft palate

A single-stage cleft palate repair is used in 97% of the centers (Table 7). Furlow Z-plasty (34.8%), pushback palatoplasty (30.3%), and intravelar veloplasty (20.4%) were the most commonly used single-stage techniques. Thirteen percent of the surgeons employed a two-stage repair in at least some cases in their practices. When a two-stage repair is employed, the vomer flap is most frequently used in the first stage (53.8%) and an intravelar veloplasty in the second stage (50%).

Forty percent of the centers reported performing Furlow Z-plasty for treatment of submucus clefts before the age of 2 years, whereas 35% of the respondents stated that they would wait until the patient was more mature (see Table 7). After the age of 2 years, the most frequent procedure employed for repair was Z-plasty (60.4%). Alternative procedures include intervelar veloplasty (17.9%) and pharyngeal flaps (12.3%).

Velopharyngeal incompetence

Speech therapy is started at an average age of 23.7 months (Table 8). The two methods for diagnosing velopharyngeal incompetence (VPI) were video nasopharyngoscopy (79.4%) and videofluoroscopy (20.6%). Eighty-one percent of the surgeons reported that lateral pharyngeal wall motion was the single most important determinant with regard to surgical planning. Palatal motion and the size of the

Table 6
Cleft nose management

Alar repositioning at time of lip repair	88.3%
Age at independent alar repositioning (%)	
4 y	45.4
5 y	27.3
6 y	18.2
>6 y	9

Table 7
Cleft palate management

Single stage	97.1%
Single-stage method (%)	
Furlow Z-plasty	34.8
Pushback technique	30.3
IVV	20.4
Two-flap technique	14.4
First stage of two-stage (%)	
Vomer	53.8
Pushback technique	23.1
IVV	15.4
Furlow Z-plasty	7.7
Second stage of two-stage (%)	
IVV	50
Pushback technique	25
Furlow Z-plasty	25
Treatment of SMC <2 y (%)	
Furlow Z-plasty	40.8
Observation	35.0
Intervelar veloplasty	18.4
Pushback technique	5.8
Treatment of SMC >2 y (%)	
Furlow Z-plasty	60.4
Intervelar veloplasty	17.9
Pharyngeal flap	12.3
Pushback technique	4.7
Observation	2.8
Levator sling	1.9

Abbreviations: IVV, intravelar veloplasty; SMC, submucus cleft.

defect were reported by the respondents as secondary determinants. The minimum age for surgical correction is reported as 4.1 years. Palatoplasty was used most frequently to address VPI (65.5%); pharyngeal flaps were employed by 34.5%.

Miscellaneous

Pressure equalization (PE) tubes are inserted at less than 3 months of age in 12.5% of the cleft centers, between 3 and 6 months in 54.2% of the centers,

Table 8
VPI management

Age at start of speech therapy	23.7 mo
VPI diagnosis method (%)	
Video nasopharygoscopy	79.4
Video Fluoroscopy	20.6
Age at VPI surgery	4.1 y
VPI method (%)	
Palatoplasty	65.5
Pharyngeal flap	34.5

Table 9
Miscellaneous

Age at PE tubes (%)	
<3 mo	12.5
3–6 mo	54.2
7–12 mo	31.7
>12 mo	1.6
Pierre Robin affects treatment	74.5%
Swallowing difficulty observed	63.8%

and between 7 and 12 months in 31.7% of the centers (Table 9). Very few patients receive PE tubes after the age of 1 year. These data suggest that a fair number of patients are getting PE tubes at the time of their initial lip repair (3–6 months). Seventy-four percent of the surgeons state that the Pierre Robin Sequence affects the timing of their cleft surgery. Sixty-three percent of the surgeons note that cleft patients have upper-aerodigestive-tract motor abnormalities that manifest as swallowing difficulties.

Discussion

The majority of the centers that responded to this study report using presurgical appliances. Most of these centers use the nasoalveolar passive molding approach. The percentage of centers reporting the use of NAM remains virtually the same in comparison with the results from the past survey (62%, 6 years ago) and represents an increase over the 48.3% usage reported in the Eurocleft Project. A cautionary note is in order with regard to comparison of the authors' data with those of the Eurocleft Project. The authors' percentages represent a proportion of the centers responding to the study, whereas the Eurocleft Project percentages represent a proportion of the individual patients included in the study project. Nonetheless, in broad terms, the comparisons help place the authors' results in the context of others' findings.

The present survey reflects a significant use of the Latham appliance by cleft centers and reflects an increase in reported usage over the past survey (5% usage, 6 years ago). The current survey unfortunately does not provide additional information that might help explain this dramatic change.

Lip adhesion is employed by just under half of the centers responding, but the overwhelming majority report using it in very few patients. Although the presence of a wide cleft is the primary reason given for the use of lip adhesion, both poor compliance with the appliance and the inability to obtain an appliance were also provided as frequent reasons for the procedure, suggesting that many centers view lip

adhesion as a second-line therapy for the wide cleft. It should be noted that a few centers reported the use of lip adhesion in all patients; centers that reported the universal use of lip adhesion did so generally for bilateral cleft patients.

Taken together, the data from the present study suggest that lip adhesion is certainly not a frequent procedure on a patient-by-patient basis. This result is consistent with those of the Eurocleft Project, which found that lip adhesion is used as a primary procedure in only 4% of patients. Compared with the past survey, this one appears to reveal a sizable decrement in the number of patients undergoing lip adhesion: 6 years ago, 89% of centers reported addressing the wide unilateral cleft with lip adhesion followed by rotation advancement.

The present study demonstrates that the majority of unilateral and bilateral cleft lips are repaired by a rotation-advancement method. This finding is consistent with the previous survey and the Eurocleft Project, which report usage rates between 50% and 89% and 50% and 62.2%, respectively. Many of the respondents in the authors' study specifically reported the use of the Millard rotation-advancement technique, but what is even more interesting is that a significant number of respondents reported using later adaptations of the original Millard technique, such as the Mulliken technique. This development is most evident in the responses regarding the repair of bilateral clefts and suggests a possible evolution in the approach to cleft care.

The present study sought significantly more information about the treatment of cleft nose deformity than did the previous survey or the Eurocleft Project, rendering a meaningful comparison impossible. Nonetheless, it should be pointed out once more that the overwhelming majority of centers do some type of alar repositioning at the time of the definitive lip repair. If alar repositioning is not performed initially, it is most frequently performed at 4 or 5 years of age; these ages are consistent with the previous study.

Unfortunately, the design of the survey does not permit discussion of the timing of palatal repair or of the number of centers that combine the repair of palatal components with the lip repair. An overwhelming majority of the centers perform a one-stage palatal repair. This figure represents a possible difference from the Eurocleft findings, which show that roughly half (51.3%) of the patients undergo one-stage soft and hard palate repair at various times, either in isolation or in combination with lip procedures. Another notable finding in the present study is the shift to the Furlow technique as the most frequently used procedure for palatal closure in a single stage. The Furlow technique is still not used in the majority of patients, as a wide variety of procedures was reported in the current study. Nonetheless, there appears to be a shift away from push-back-type techniques, which were reported as the most commonly used method in the survey 6 years ago. The rise in prominence of the Furlow techniques is also demonstrated in the results pertaining to the care of the submucus cleft. When a two-stage procedure is indicated, the most frequent sequence is a vomer flap followed by intervelar veloplasty.

The diagnosis of VPI continues to be confirmed with video nasopharyngoscopy and videofluoroscopy. Lateral wall motion, followed by palatal motion, is the most significant determinant for management.

Summary

The present study presents a contemporary (2004) survey of the methods and timing used in the care of cleft patients. The results are compared, when possible, with those of a similar study published by the lead author in 1998 and with those of the Eurocleft Project that took place from 1996 to 2000. Although very little uniformity is seen in the care of cleft patients, this comparison demonstrates a significant degree of agreement on many aspects of cleft care. The use of presurgical orthopedic appliances, generally of the NAM type, is predominant. The use of rotation advancement maintains its predominance in the repair of the cleft lip and is generally accompanied by alar repositioning. The area of greatest variation and diversity is the care of the palate, where the Furlow technique has become a frequently used procedure. Comparison of the results of this study with the findings of the previous two demonstrates a continuing process of adaptation and evolution in the field of cleft lip and palate surgery.

References

[1] Stal S, Klebuc M, Taylor T, Spira M, Edwards M. Algorithms for the treatment of cleft lip and palate. Clin Plast Surg 1998;25(4):493–507.

[2] European Commission. Directorate-General XII, Science, Research, and Development. The Eurocleft Project 1996–2000. Washington, DC: IOS Press; 2000.

[3] Grayson BH, Santiago PE, Brecht LE, Cutting CB. Presurgical nasoalveolar molding in infants with cleft lip and palate. Cleft Palate Craniofac J 1999;36(6): 486–98.

[4] Latham RA, Kusy RP, Georgiade NG. An extraorally activated expansion appliance for cleft palate infants. Cleft Palate J 1976;13:253–61.

[5] Millard Jr DR. Cleft craft: the unilateral deformity, Vol. 1. Boston: Little Brown; 1976. p. 210.

[6] Mohler LR. Unilateral cleft lip repair. Plast Reconstr Surg 1986;80(4):511–6.

[7] Mulliken JB. Repair of the bilateral complete cleft lip and nasal deformity: state of the art. Cleft Palate Craniofac J 2000;37:342–7.

[8] Akguner M, Barutcu A, Karaca C. Adolescent growth patterns of the bony and cartilaginous framework of the nose: a cephalometric study. Ann Plast Surg 1998;41: 66–9.

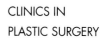

CLINICS IN
PLASTIC SURGERY

Clin Plastic Surg 32 (2005) 25 – 34

Separation of craniopagus conjoined twins: an evolution in thought

David A. Staffenberg, MD[a,b,]*, James T. Goodrich, MD, PhD[a,b]

[a]*Children's Hospital at Montefiore, Montefiore Medical Center, 3415 Bainbridge Avenue, Bronx, NY 10467, USA*
[b]*Albert Einstein College of Medicine, 1300 Morris Park Avenue, Bronx, NY 10461, USA*

Craniopagus twins occur in about 2% of conjoined twins. In craniopagus cases, the union can occur anywhere on the cranial vault but, by definition, does not involve the foramen magnum, face, vertebrae, or base of the skull. The thorax and abdomen are completely separate. The junction of the conjoined twins is rarely symmetric and can involve any part of the meninges, venous sinuses, and cortex. Axial and rotational orientation is variable. Each of these factors can influence the development, distortion, deformation, and displacement of the brain, the meninges, and the vascular system, as well as the prognosis after surgical separation.

Four types of conjoined twins are joined at the head: (1) *craniopagus* twins are joined only in the calvarium; (2) *cephalopagus* twins are joined ventrally, from the top of the head down to the umbilicus; (3) *parapagus diprosopus* twins are joined laterally with two faces on one head but share only one body;
(4) *rachipagus* twins are joined dorsally along the vertebral column, occasionally involving the occiput.

The female-to-male ratio in craniopagus twins is about 4:1, which is similar to the ratio for other types of conjoined twins. Other anomalies that have been reported are congenital heart disease, cleft lip, cleft palate, supernumerary thumbs, extrophy of the cloaca and absence of the entire urinary tract, bladder extrophy, absence of anus and vagina, and imperforate anus [1].

Classification

The simplest method of classification of craniopagus twins refers to the site of junction: *frontal, temporal, parietal, occipital,* or combinations of these. O'Connell [1] has suggested the use of the terms *partial* and *total* to describe the degree of junction. He further divides cases into types I, II, and III to indicate whether the twins are facing in the same or opposite directions or whether their axes are perpendicular to each other. The authors' case represents an O'Connell type I (Fig. 1).

Winston et al [2] described a classification system based on the embryologic origin of the deepest shared structure: the surface ectoderm and cranium, the dura (ectomeninx), the leptomeninges (endomeninx), or the neuroectoderm. Todorov et al [3] correlated postoperative survival with the axial orientation of the union. They describe the acute frontal–frontal angle as being most favorable, with mortality increasing as that angle increases.

All parties involved in the staged separation have donated their care. Philanthropic support provided by the Children's Hospital at Montefiore, Montefiore Medical Center (Bronx, NY), Blythedale Children's Hospital (Valhalla, NY), Medical Modeling (Golden, CO), Voxel (Provo, UT), Hill-Rom (Batesville, IN), Mentor Corp. (Santa Barbara, CA), Children's Chance (Waterbury, CT), Knightsbridge International (West Hills, CA), Philippine Airlines Foundation (Manila, Philippines), and Hanger Prosthetics and Orthotics (Farmingdale, NY).

* Corresponding author. Children's Hospital at Montefiore, 3415 Bainbridge Avenue, Bronx, NY 10467.

E-mail address: dstaffen@montefiore.org
(D.A. Staffenberg).

0094-1298/05/$ – see front matter © 2005 Elsevier Inc. All rights reserved.
doi:10.1016/j.cps.2004.09.002

plasticsurgery.theclinics.com

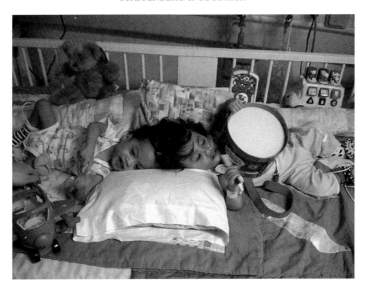

Fig. 1. Craniopagus twins; Twin A on left. (Courtesy of Montefiore Medical Center/Alice Attie; with permission.)

Spencer [4] points out that each of these systems has merit, but they fail to take into account the anatomy of the underlying dural venous sinuses. She suggests that it is the specific anatomy of these vessels that "doom[s] the vast majority of these infants to the wretched life of intact conjoined twins or the significant risk of death or serious neurologic impairment following surgical separation."

The configuration of the dural sinuses appears to be influenced by three factors. (1) The farther the site of union is from the nasion and midline and the closer to the inion, the more likely is the involvement of the dural sinuses. (2) The larger the plane of intersection, the greater is the probability that the sinuses and cortical surfaces will be fused. (3) The greater the rotation and the more obtuse the angulation from the frontal area, the more likely the sinuses and cerebral hemispheres are to be involved. Likewise, the larger the area of confluence of the scalps, the greater the soft tissue requirement for reconstruction.

The dural sinuses are not true veins; they do not contain valves, muscles, or fibrous walls and are therefore very fragile. The sinuses are not movable within the surrounding tissue.

The location of the sinuses in the conjoined area may be hard to predict, and the direction of blood flow is variable. When the twins are joined vertex-to-vertex, the falx cerebri does not form and the superior sagittal sinus cannot develop. Its analogue forms around the periphery of the conjoined plane in a fold of dura. This shared dural ring, or shelf, contains a venous sinus that can be either completely or partially circumferential and may also form a "venous lake." Each twin will have veins draining into this sinus. Extracranial arteries are an important consideration when planning skin flaps. It is rare that the union of the calvaria affects the intracranial arteries.

Winston [2] points out that adequate support must be provided to avoid gravitational forces on the brains during separation surgery. The possibility of air embolism is of concern during separation as well. Any external pressure on the jugular veins must be carefully avoided, because this can increase venous pressure and consequently bleeding and cerebral edema. The relative position of the twins on induction of anesthesia and surgery may cause some degree of "transfusion" from one twin to the other. The issue of adrenal dominance is important in any kind of conjoined twinning; the twin with adrenal suppression may require steroid supplementation preoperatively, intraoperatively, and postoperatively [5].

Surgical history

The first attempt at separation of craniopagus recorded in the twentieth century involved 12-day-old infants with parietal union; neither survived this attempt [6]. The first survival recorded was of 14-month-old males with a large parietal union, a shared sinus in a semicircular dural shelf, and a single confluence. Massive hemorrhage occurred when the veins were divided. The first twin died 34 days after surgery; the second survived with a temporary hemiparesis but died of complications of hydrocephalus at 11 years of age [7]. The first recorded survival of both twins was in a set of 7-month-old girls with minimal parietal union. The authors describe a thin sheet of bone across the plane of union. The twins shared a 5-mm segment of the superior sagittal sinus. One twin is reported to have survived intact in spite of massive hemorrhage, but the other suffered severe neurologic injury. Interestingly, the neurologically impaired twin donated a kidney to her sister 28 years later [4,8].

Efforts have been made to alter the size and angulation of the union. Wolfowitz et al [9] successfully increased the angle of union between a set of frontoparietal twins in an effort to increase the surgical exposure. In another case, a metal band was placed circumferentially around the plane of junction but required removal when the twins developed seizures [10]. In yet another set of craniopagus conjoined twins, constriction by a plastic ring was abandoned when the resulting ulcer became infected [11]. An adjustable pneumatic cuff was placed around another set of twins. The bridge was decreased by 10%, preventing subsequent growth of the conjoined area, but the 5-month-old males with a minimal occipitoparietal union died of massive hemorrhage in the operating room [12]. In a German case with extensive parietal union, a circular nylon band was used unsuccessfully [13].

In her review of this topic, Spencer [4] notes that the most important data to obtain before surgery concern the location and character of the dural sinuses. It is clear that division of the veins draining into the dural sinus can result in elevated venous pressure and venous infarcts. In addition, such elevation in venous pressure may result in significant cerebral edema, making reconstruction more difficult. Cardiopulmonary bypass, hypothermia, intraluminal shunting, and circulatory arrest with division and reconstruction of the major sinuses have led to minimal success [14].

A set of craniopagus conjoined twins was separated in stages with gradual closure of a bridging vein. To accomplish this, a screw clamp with an exteriorized stem was used over several days gradually to occlude a short bridging vein between superior sagittal sinuses. This method led to a successful separation, but no long-term follow-up was reported [15].

Continued advances in anesthesia techniques and critical care have improved the chances of survival in craniopagus separation. Insertion of tissue expanders followed by a lengthy separation surgery was performed in a set of Guatemalan female craniopagus twins (University of California, Los Angeles), and a similar technique was used to separate a pair of male twins from Egypt. In the latter set, an innovative rotating table was fabricated to allow the twins to be rotated along their axis in unison. In these cases, each twin survived, but there were notable neurologic deficits more than 6 months after each separation.

A set of 29-year-old Iranian women joined temporoparietally hemorrhaged to death during their attempted separation. Although medical models were used and the surgeons had the advantage of many recent technological innovations, they noted that, after hours of surgery to divide the other veins, the final bridging vein was enormously dilated and there was significant venous engorgement. This hypertension is probably due to the acute change in venous pathways.

An evolution of thought

A careful review of personal communications and the literature has convinced the authors that a prolonged operation to ligate and divide the bridging veins in these cases leads to unavoidable venous hypertension and circulatory compromise of the brain. Plastic surgical principles lead one to consider staged division of venous tributaries to encourage the development of venous collaterals and the resulting diversion of drainage [16].

Although previously attempted staged techniques have had mixed results, the authors believe that the stages must be timed so that complete recovery is allowed to ensue between them. These breaks between surgical stages allow for occupational and physical therapy and nutritional support and facilitate the desired vascular changes. A staged approach enables the patients to be exposed to general anesthetics for shorter periods of time, to require fewer intravenous fluids and transfusion products, and to have less bleeding and cerebral edema. Although the skin flaps must be completely designed from the beginning of the staged procedures, elevating the flaps for each stage offers the delay phenomenon to the skin flaps. Perhaps the most important benefit of the staged procedure is that it allows the bridging veins to be divided sequentially, thereby promoting the improvement of collateral venous drainage. The authors hypothesize that the improvement in venous drainage, together with the previously discussed advantages, will improve the neurologic outcome. At the final stage, during separation, improved venous drainage and shorter surgical time before separation

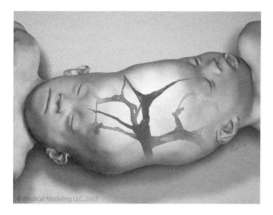

Fig. 2. Illustration showing skin envelope with conjoined venous system superimposed from initial CT data; Twin A on right. (Courtesy of Montefiore Medical Center and Medical Modeling [Golden, Colorado]; with permission.)

will result in reduced cerebral edema, making dura and scalp reconstruction less complicated.

Case review

On April 21, 2002, a 29-year-old woman in the Philippines gave birth to a set of male craniopagus twins by cesarean section. A level-2 ultrasound had diagnosed the condition; termination of the pregnancy was offered but was rejected because of religious conviction. The mother desired separation for the twins, and a work-up was obtained (Fig. 1).

During intubation for MRI and CT studies, twin A suffered aspiration pneumonia twice. Further efforts

at work-up were abandoned, and transfer to the Children's Hospital at Montefiore was arranged. Arrangements were made to augment the twins' nutrition and provide pulmonary care and intensive occupational and physical therapy at Blythedale Children's Hospital in Valhalla, New York. The authors have a long-standing relationship with Blythedale, a rehabilitation center that does not provide acute care.

On arrival in New York, the twins presented evidence of failure to thrive, and twin A, much smaller than twin B, was noted to have severe hypertension and tachycardia. Antihypertensive medication was prescribed. Urine output was also noted to be greater in twin A.

Craniofacial CT with three-dimensional reconstruction was obtained, as well as MRI and magnetic resonance venography (MRV). Data from these studies were used to obtain diagrams and clear stereolithographic models (Medical Modeling, Golden, Colorado) of the shared venous system within the conjoined skulls (Fig. 2). In addition, a three-dimensional model of the skin envelope was obtained (Medical Modeling, Golden, Colorado). This model is quite useful to the plastic surgeon, and a pencil can be used to design skin flaps (Fig. 3).

Scalp flaps were designed to maximize the twins' blood supply and avoid suture lines over the vertex of the scalp once they were separated. A sinusoidal pattern was designed to accomplish this goal.

Flaps were designed to extend toward the opposite twin's right ear, leaving the incisions to resemble a sinusoidal curve around the conjoined scalp. Because the twins' interaxial angle was less than 180° (see Fig. 3), one twin would have a shorter flap. Although tissue expansion would be used, the twin who was expected to have the larger

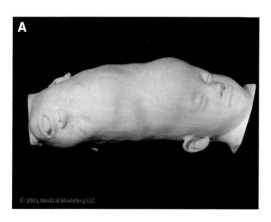

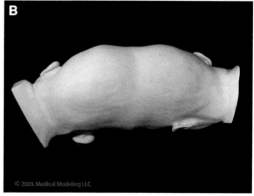

Fig. 3. Three-dimensional model fabricated from CT data. (*A*) Anterior view; Twin A on left. (*B*) Posterior view; Twin A on right. (Courtesy of Montefiore Medical Center and Medical Modeling [Golden, Colorado]; with permission.)

dural defect and patch was given the longer flap. It was crucial to identify this twin before the first stage of separation.

Craniofacial CT and MRI/MRV studies were also used to generate holograms (Voxel, Provo, Utah). To the authors' knowledge, this is the first time holographic images have been used in the separation of conjoined twins (Fig. 4).

When a single-staged separation of craniopagus twins is planned, tissue expansion can be performed on intact scalp without previous surgery, thereby minimizing the risks associated with tissue expansion

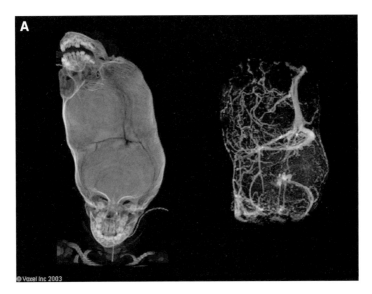

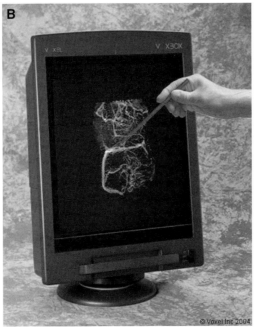

Fig. 4. (*A*) Hologram from CT data on left and MRV data on right (these can be overlaid). (*B*) Holograms projected in front of viewbox. (Courtesy of Montefiore Medical Center and Voxel [Provo, Utah]; with permission.)

(eg, exposure and infection) [17]. During the separation, however, the expanders require removal, and the expanded scalp undergoes a degree of retraction during the hours of neurosurgery required to separate the twins in a single-staged separation. By contrast, tissue expansion during a multiple-staged separation is more complicated. The requirement of performing tissue expansion after previous stages, with healing scars and manipulated tissue, is a challenge unique to the staged approach. In each of the stages, exposure is provided through the previously designed flaps, and the craniotomies are kept as narrow as possible, overlying the conjoined plane. Tissue expansion was planned at each stage, replacing the expanders each time with a larger size. The authors believed that the size of the expanders would need to increase gradually, as the healing scars grew longer with each stage.

Multiple dental caries were noted on examination. These represented possible sources of bacteremia, and multiple extractions were performed under general anesthesia. From that point on, anesthesiologists were dedicated to the continued care of each specific twin throughout his various stages. The authors' dedicated craniofacial surgery scrub technicians and circulating nurses made the same commitment.

Stage 1

On October 20, 2003, stage 1 was performed. Intraoperative navigation was used (Stryker Corp., Kalamazoo, MI). The conjoined twins were positioned supine, and the forehead was opened along the planned incision line, exposing the shared frontal bone. A frontal craniotomy was performed, and dura was divided adjacent to the line of fusion on the side of twin B. A circumferential "shelf" of dura was seen. This shelf was the dura enveloping the circumferential sinus, which would ultimately be left with twin A. Brains were seen to be separate. A large anterior bridging vein in twin B was divided at this stage (Fig. 5). A silastic sheet was placed between the brains to avoid adhesions. Dura was repaired, and the craniotomy was closed with titanium miniplates. The authors typically use resorbable fixation in their pediatric craniofacial work, but in this case, because hardware would need to be removed during the final separation, they applied titanium hardware. One-hundred-milliliter tissue expanders (Inamed, Santa Barbara, California) were then placed adjacent to the craniotomy, and the scalp was closed in layers.

Subgaleal fluid leaked from the suture lines 10 days postoperatively, and worsening fevers led to

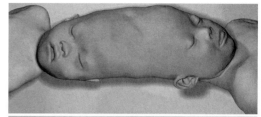
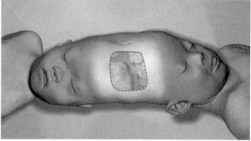
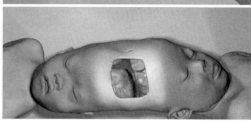

Fig. 5. Note orientation and large bridging vein that was ligated (clipped) and divided, leaving the circumferential venous sinus with twin A on left. (Courtesy of Montefiore Medical Center and Medical Modeling [Golden, Colorado]; with permission.)

removal of the tissue expanders. Otherwise, recovery was uncomplicated.

Stage 2

On November 24, 2003, the twins returned to the operating room for the second stage. The skin incision was lengthened toward the left ear of twin A and farther along to the occipital area, allowing the second craniotomy to be performed. Bridging veins were temporarily clamped on twin B's side of the circumferential sinus. No sign of cortical edema was observed, so these veins were ligated and divided (Fig. 6). The previously placed silastic sheet was replaced. Closure was performed after placement of new tissue expanders. The tissue expanders were removed 14 days later for similar reasons to those used in the first stage. At this point, the authors believed that tissue expansion should be performed

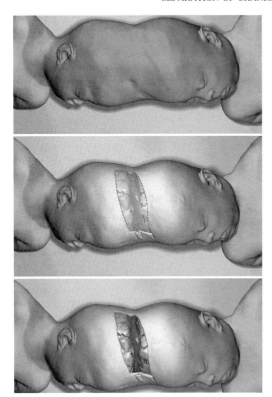

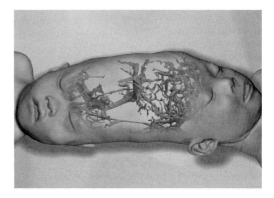

Fig. 7. Increased quality of venous collaterals; Twin B on left. (Courtesy of Montefiore Medical Center and Medical Modeling [Golden, Colorado]; with permission.)

Fig. 6. Note orientation and bridging veins that were ligated (clipped) and divided, leaving the circumferential venous sinus with twin A on left. (Courtesy of Montefiore Medical Center and Medical Modeling [Golden, Colorado]; with permission.)

separately from the craniotomies, because of the expected cerebrospinal fluid leaks into the surgical site.

Stage 3

New CT scans and MRI/MRV were obtained, and on February 20, 2004, the third stage of the twins' vascular separation was performed. CT and MRI/MRV studies were repeated between stages to confirm the development of the needed venous collaterals (Fig. 7). From the first procedure, timing between stages was judged subjectively with attention to the twins' progress in physical therapy as well as their soft tissue healing. No predetermined schedule was used.

The twins were placed in prone position, and the incision was lengthened along its predesigned path and an occipital craniotomy performed. Vessels were addressed in similar fashion, and closure was performed (Fig. 8).

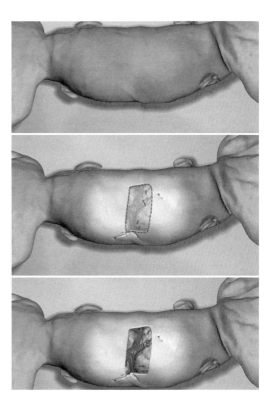

Fig. 8. Note orientation and bridging veins that were ligated (clipped) and divided, leaving the circumferential venous sinus with twin A on left. (Courtesy of Montefiore Medical Center and Medical Modeling [Golden, Colorado]; with permission.)

Tissue expanders were placed 8 weeks before the twins' expected separation surgery. Expanders were placed over each left ear, through separate incisions behind the ears, in areas where no previous operations had been performed. Subcutaneous ports were placed behind the earlobes, and expansion was begun 3 weeks after placement.

Stage 4

Final separation surgery was perfomed on August 4, 2004, 9.5 months after the first stage. Placement of the tissue expanders above the ears allowed them to remain in place while the separation was performed. Continued circumferential dissection and division of the remaining dura and veins facilitated their separation in a controlled fashion. Despite abundant preoperative imaging, a shared posterior temporal lobe was encountered and was divided according to its vascular pattern (Fig. 9).

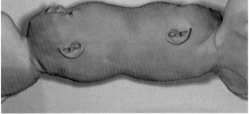
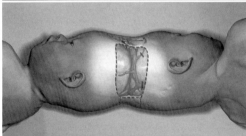
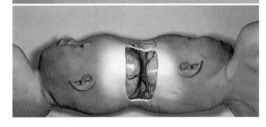

Fig. 9. Note orientation and bridging veins that were ligated (clipped) and divided, leaving the circumferential venous sinus with twin A on left. (Courtesy of Montefiore Medical Center and Medical Modeling [Golden, Colorado]; with permission.)

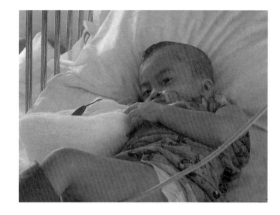

Fig. 10. Twin B on postoperative day 14; he managed to remove his entire head dressing.

Once the twins were separated, the operating tables were rotated approximately 30° to allow teams to work side by side. This rotation was thought to require the least amount of movement in the operating room (tables pivoted on their pedestals, so anesthesia teams did not need to move) and therefore to be the safest maneuver. Durasis (Cook Biotech, West Lafayette, Indiana) was used to replace missing dura; tissue expanders were removed and scalp flaps closed. Twin B underwent complete primary closure over the large dural graft, while Alloderm (LifeCell, Branchburg, New Jersey) was placed over the native dura over the right ear of Twin A.

Through all stages of surgery, the twins shared 4175 cm^3 of packed red blood cells. No drains or primary shunts were used during the final separation. The twins were lightly sedated until their extubation, which occurred on postoperative day 3 for twin B and postoperative day 4 for twin A. Prophylactic phenobarbital was used for each procedure. As of their

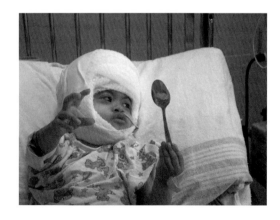

Fig. 11. Twin A on postoperative day 14.

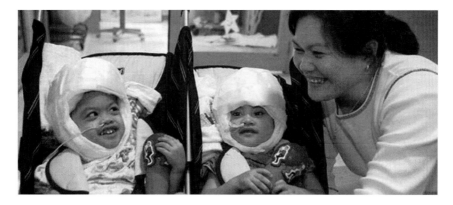

Fig. 12. The separated twins on postoperative day 25; Twin A on left. (Courtesy of Montefiore Medical Center; with permission.)

discharge from the hospital 3.5 weeks postoperatively, neither twin has developed hydrocephalus. Both twins are neurologically intact, interactive, and playful; they have begun to eat baby food. Twin A's antihypertensive medications were discontinued 1 week after surgery. Wounds are healing without evidence of cerebrospinal fluid leak (Fig. 10).

At the time of this writing, the twins have been discharged to Blythedale Children's Hospital to continue speech and feeding therapy, as well as occupational and physical therapy. As healing progresses, additional scalp flap advancement will provide complete scalp coverage in twin A; calvarial vault reconstruction in each twin will follow (see Fig. 10; Figs. 11 and 12).

Discussion

Craniopagus conjoined twins are a rare entity. Advances in anesthesia and critical care management have resulted in survival of both twins in several cases. Among surviving twins, neurologic injury has been common in reported cases of O'Connell type-I twins. To the authors' knowledge, no such twins have been able to lead independent, productive lives as a separated pair. After the authors were asked to evaluate such a pair of infants for separation, their evolution in thought began with the more commonly performed single-staged neurosurgical separation. A review of the available literature made clear that dividing the shared veins in a single stage was a likely source of brain injury. Furthermore, the authors' experience in craniofacial surgery indicates that patients, especially infants and children, recover more easily when procedures are done expeditiously.

The literature includes some cases separated in stages, but these stages were close together, and morbidity and mortality appear to have been essentially unchanged. We became convinced that a carefully planned multiple-staged separation could allow for the desired outcome only if the patients were allowed appropriate recovery time between stages. After each stage, the authors would not be able to predict the amount of time needed for recovery, but their team was committed to close observation and an open-ended schedule.

With the preservation of neurologic function as their prime goal, the authors discovered the difficulties of a staged separation. Tissue expansion has higher morbidity when performed at the same time as a craniotomy. Vascular clips are needed on the edges of the dura, which then compromise a water-tight closure, leading to increased amounts of fluid around the tissue expanders. The limited area around the heads makes it difficult to place the expanders in a site where they are not exposed to this fluid and to the resulting risk of infection and exposure. Based on their experience, the authors believe that expansion should be done as an isolated procedure before the final stage. Additional issues may arise as the soft tissue envelope is repeatedly elevated, leading to some trauma. But this problem may be countered by a delay phenomenon, as the flaps are elevated and returned to their original position, only to be used at a later stage.

Separation surgery in multiple stages has the potential to reduce exposure to general anesthesia, bleeding, use of intravenous fluids, transfusion requirement, cerebral edema, and fatigue in the surgical team. The venous drainage between twins may be analogized to automobile traffic in New York City.

In a single-staged separation, all of the bridging veins are ligated and divided during the course of surgery. This process may be likened to closing off all the cross-streets in midtown at the same time, which would surely lead to "gridlock": traffic would come to a stop. The circulatory equivalent in the brain is a frightening thought. However, if those same cross-streets were closed off gradually, drivers would learn to use alternate routes to get to their destinations; existing roadways could be employed, and New York City would not need to build new roads. In like manner, the authors' surgical procedure encourages venous collaterals in each brain to mature gradually to handle the needed increase in flow.

To plastic surgeons, this analogy and the authors' experience with this separation may be seen as particularly gratifying, because we are constantly concerned with manipulating living tissue to maintain or improve function. At the time of writing, 25 days after their final separation surgery, the twins have been transferred from the pediatric intensive care unit at the Children's Hospital at Montefiore to resume their rehabilitation at Blythedale Children's Hospital. No detectable neurologic deficits were reported by the authors' neurology colleagues who received them.

References

[1] O'Connell JEA. Craniopagus twins: surgical anatomy and embryology and their implications. J Neurol Neurosurg Psychiatry 1976;39:1–22.

[2] Winston KR, Rockoff MA, Mulliken JB, et al. Surgical division of craniopagi. Neurosurgery 1987;21:782–91.

[3] Todorov AB, Cohen KI, Spilotro V, Landau E. Craniopagus twins. J Neurol Neurosurg Psychiatry 1974;37: 1291–8.

[4] Spencer R. Conjoined twins: developmental malformations and clinical implications. Baltimore (MD): Johns Hopkins University Press; 2003.

[5] Aird I, Hamilton WJ, Wijthoff JPS, Lord JM. The surgery of conjoined twins. Proc R Soc Med 1954;47: 681–8.

[6] Cameron HC. A craniopagus. Lancet 1928;1:284–5.

[7] Grossman HJ, Sugar O, Greeley PW, Sadove MS. Surgical separation in craniopagus. JAMA 1953;153: 201–7.

[8] Voris HC, Slaughter WB, Christian JR, Cayia ER. Successful separation of craniopagus twins. J Neurosurg 1957;14:548–60.

[9] Wolfowitz J, Kerr EM, Levin SE, et al. Separation of craniopagus. S Afr Med J 1968;42:412–24.

[10] Wong KC, Ohmura A, Roberts TH, et al. Anesthetic management for separation of craniopagus twins. Anesth Analg 1980;59:883–6.

[11] O'Neill Jr JA, Holcomb III GW, Schnaufer L, et al. Surgical experience with 13 conjoined twins. Ann Surg 1988;208:299–312.

[12] Gaist G, Piazza G, Galassi E, et al. Craniopagus twins: an unsuccessful separation and a clinical review of the entity. Childs Nerv Syst 1987;3:327–33.

[13] Aird I. Conjoined twins: further observations. BMJ 1959;1:1313–5.

[14] Cameron DE, Reitz BA, Carson BS, et al. Separation of craniopagus Siamese twins using cardiopulmonary bypass and hypothermic circulatory arrest. J Thorac Cardiovasc Surg 1989;98:961–7.

[15] Drummond G, Scott P, Mackay D, Lipschitz R. Separation of the Baragwanath craniopagus twins. Br J Plast Surg 1991;44:49–52.

[16] Roberts TS. Cranial venous abnormalities in craniopagus twins. In: Kapp JP, Schmidek HH, editors. The cerebral venous system and its disorders. Orlando (FL): Grune & Stratton; 1984. p. 355–71.

[17] Zubowicz VN, Ricketts R. Use of skin expanders in separation of conjoined twins. Ann Plast Surg 1988; 20:272–6.

Clin Plastic Surg 32 (2005) 35 – 44

CLINICS IN
PLASTIC SURGERY

Tissue expansion in pediatric patients

Roxana Rivera, MD, John LoGiudice, MD, Arun K. Gosain, MD*

Department of Plastic Surgery, Medical College of Wisconsin, 9200 West Wisconsin Avenue, Milwaukee, WI 53226, USA

Tissue expansion has become a well-recognized technique for reconstructing a wide variety of skin and soft tissue defects. Its application in the pediatric population has allowed the plastic surgeon to achieve functional and aesthetic goals that were previously unobtainable. This technique can be applied to a variety of reconstructive problems, including the management of giant congenital nevi and the secondary reconstruction of extensive burn scars, making possible the use of sensate tissue of similar color, texture, thickness, and hair-bearing characteristics to resurface the affected areas. However, when using tissue expanders, one must be prepared for complications, because they are inherent in a process in which skin is expanded by the repeated filling of an implanted foreign body. Complication rates increase when serial expansion of the same tissues is performed repeatedly, or if expanders are placed in the lower extremities. Outcomes are dependent on thorough preoperative planning, parent and patient teaching, meticulous technique, close follow-up, and patient compliance.

The authors review the use of tissue expansion in the pediatric population, with particular emphasis on indications, operative technique, and regional considerations. They also address concerns that have been expressed about the complications associated with this technique.

Historical overview

The expansion of skin was first reported in 1957 by Neumann [1], who used a rubber balloon with an external port in the reconstruction of a traumatic ear defect. The periauricular skin was serially expanded over a four-month period without extrusion or infection. This procedure was ignored until 1976, when Radovan [2] presented his experience with breast reconstruction. Austad and Rose [3] followed with their description of a self-inflating expander in 1982. The first description of tissue expansion in the pediatric population was in 1983 by Argenta et al [4], who used it in the treatment of neck contractures in burn patients.

Characteristics of expanded tissue

Both animal and human studies have documented histologic changes in soft tissue undergoing expansion. Mechanical force on skin influences numerous aspects of cellular architecture and function, including cytoskeleton structure, extracellular matrix, enzyme activity, second-messenger systems, and ion channel activity [5,6]. Expansion in a guinea pig model demonstrated significant thickening of the epidermis as early as 1 week after the start of the procedure. By contrast, the dermis thins during expansion. Austad et al [7] concluded that the epidermis exhibits increased mitotic activity soon after expansion begins, with a spike in activity 7 days later. Such mitotic activity is not present in the dermis. These phenomena have been observed in other animal models, as well as in humans [8,9].

In human studies, it does not appear that expander volume or anatomic location has any influence on dermal thickness. No histologic differences appear to distinguish adults undergoing expansion from children. Light microscopy reveals flattening of the rete ridges as well as epidermal thickening. Skin appendages demonstrate no histologic changes during

* Corresponding author.
E-mail address: gosain@mcw.edu (A.K. Gosain).

0094-1298/05/$ – see front matter © 2005 Elsevier Inc. All rights reserved.
doi:10.1016/j.cps.2004.08.001

expansion. Capillaries in the papillary dermis are dilated on light microscopy. Electron microscopy reveals longer and thicker elastic fibers and active fibroblasts with an abundance of rough endoplasmic reticulum [9].

Subcutaneous tissue displays significant fat atrophy with flattening of adipocytes. Muscle under expansion also atrophies and can be replaced by fibrous tissue. Expander capsule thickness does not seem to be related to expander volume, location, or patient age [9].

Samples of human skin taken some time after completion of expansion and removal of the expander showed a reversal in the epidermal thickening and dermal thinning that occurred with expansion. Blood vessels of the skin and subcutaneous tissue were normal in size and number [9].

Indications for tissue expansion in pediatric plastic surgery

Initially described in the modern literature as a modality for ear reconstruction, tissue expansion is now used for a variety of clinical problems [10–15]. Burn scars that would otherwise have been left untreated can now be addressed regardless of size, reducing the physical and emotional morbidity of such wounds [16]. Giant congenital nevi can be treated in a satisfactory manner with single-stage or serial expansion and excision, regardless of location and size. This technique has replaced partial excision and dermabrasion and helped to eliminate some of the risks that may accompany incomplete excision of such premalignant lesions [17,18]. Ideally, expansion is begun in the early months of life to avoid the peer-group pressure that develops later in childhood. Early reports warned that deformities of the craniofacial skeleton might result from expansion in infants and children, but there appears to be no permanent disturbance of growth or skeletal deformity [19,20]. It has been advocated that expanders with semirigid backing be used if there is a concern about distortion of underlying structures. In addition, expansion should be delayed until the patient is 6 to 9 months of age if molding of the cranium is evident [21].

Tissue expansion has been applied in the pediatric population in the treatment of aplasia cutis congenita, meningomyelocele, microtia, hemangioma, scrotal reconstruction, clubfoot deformity, midfacial cleft, Romberg's disease, Poland's syndrome, tumor ablation, vaginal agenesis, and Volkmann's contracture and in the reconstruction after separation of conjoined twins [20,22–24].

Expansion of soft tissue may be employed to increase the size of full-thickness skin grafts, local or regional flaps, or distant or free flaps before transfer. The advantage of harvesting expanded full-thickness skin grafts or flaps is that maximum yield is obtained with reduced donor-site morbidity. No evidence has been found of greater contraction or decreased durability of the expanded tissue when compared with a nonexpanded full-thickness graft or flap [25].

Operative technique

General considerations

Antibiotic use

Because no study has addressed this issue prospectively, the use of perioperative antibiotics should be considered on a case-by-case basis.

Choice and placement of the expander

Expanders are available in a variety of shapes, sizes, contours, and backing configurations. Expander shape and size are chosen based on the dimensions of the defect and the configuration of the surrounding normal skin. This selection process has largely been guided by the preference of the surgeon, because no data indicate that an expander of a given shape is more advantageous for placement in a given site. In some situations, a custom-designed expander may be preferable, to facilitate maximal expansion with less likelihood of donor-site morbidity. Several authors have demonstrated that employing calculations to predict the area expanded often leads to an over-estimation of actual expander yield [26,27]. Because contraction is expected, the expander should create a flap that is 30% to 50% longer than necessary when maximally filled [28].

Expanders are usually placed while the patient is under general anesthesia. Incisions for placement of the expander should be carefully planned. Consideration must be given to the advancement or rotation of the planned flap, the effects of expansion on the overlying skin, and the potential donor-site morbidity. Making straight incisions along the border of the defect should usually be avoided. Options when placing an incision include placement perpendicular to the direction of expansion and placement of a V- or U-shaped incision away from the defect [28]. If an incision must be placed near the defect, the pocket should be dissected as far from it as possible. The authors recommend a margin of 2 cm or greater from the incision to the desired expander pocket to minimize the risk of dehiscence when expansion commences. Expansion should be delayed until wound healing has progressed sufficiently, usually at least 2 weeks. When planning for a large congenital nevus that will require serial expansion, one should place the incision within the lesion, removed from the proposed expander pocket, to avoid compromising subsequent expansions [21,29].

The expander pocket should be made as close to the size of the expander as possible so as to avoid subluxation of the expander. Blunt dissection is frequently indicated to preserve the overlying vessels. This measure is especially important where longitudinal vessels are present and serial expansion will be needed [30]. Dissection is usually done over the deep fascia unless the underlying muscle is to be included in the flap. In the case of a nevus, the pocket dissection should extend to the junction of normal skin and nevus. This measure should prevent expander migration under the nevus and subsequent stretching of the nevus, while allowing the skin–nevus junction to serve as the edge of the advancement flap. In the scalp, expanders are usually placed in a subgaleal pocket.

Injection ports may be internal or external and remote or integrated into the expander. Neumann's application in 1957 employed an external port in an adult [2]. Internal ports subsequently became more popular, because this arrangement ensures a "closed" system with presumably less likelihood for port disruption and expander infection. However, this advantage has been disputed. Jackson et al [31] presented their experience with external reservoirs with only a 5.6% complication rate, which was far less than the 20% to 40% complication rate noted in many series that used internal ports. Lozano and Drucker [32] reported their experience using 34 expanders with external ports in 28 pediatric patients, most of which were placed in the head and neck. They noted a combined infection and exposure rate of 17.6%. These authors cited reduced dissection, painless port access, and earlier detection of leaks as reasons to use external ports. In reporting their experience using internal ports, Bauer et al [21] emphasized that the port should be low-profile in areas where there is potential undue pressure on the overlying skin and should be remote from the expander to ensure that the expander is not punctured when it is accessed. In planning the placement of remote ports, the surgeon must consider that the distance between the expander and the port may change when expansion commences. What appears to be an adequate distance at the time of placement may be insufficient when the expander is fully inflated.

Some authors advocate the use of drains, whereas others emphasize strict hemostasis and initial filling of the expander intraoperatively to render a drain unnecessary [21,22].

Expander inflation

Most authors start the inflation process 2 to 4 weeks after expander insertion and repeat the injections on a weekly basis. The interval and volume of expansion will vary by region and wound type. The rate of inflation of the expanders is also variable and depends on physical findings and patient comfort. Inspection of skin color (blanching), capillary refill, and simple palpation are performed when additional expansion is under consideration. Overinflation of tissue expanders beyond the manufacturer's recommended fill-capacity appears to be the norm in clinical practice [22,33]. In one clinical study, overexpansion was shown to be associated with a lower complication rate than was underexpansion [34]. In this study, an expander was inflated 3.5 times its manufacturer's stated capacity without complication. An ex vivo study of expanders from multiple vendors has shown that mean overinflation of 80 times the manufacturer's stated capacity can be achieved [35].

Following closure, a small volume of sterile saline solution is usually injected into the expander both to confirm that the system is working properly and to maintain the volume of the expander pocket during capsule formation. A capsule will begin to form very early after expander placement, and, if the expander has folded on itself or has constricted in the area occupied, the capsule will limit the surface area for expansion to less than that of the planned dissection pocket.

Expander use with flaps

Local and regional flaps should be planned according to the principles discussed earlier, with emphasis on incision placement and pocket dissection that avoid enlarging the defect. The flaps most commonly used are an advancement flap or transposition flap, or a combination of the two. Selecting the size of the expander may not be a straightforward process, because of the difficulty of calculating actual flap gain [26,27]. Different techniques have been proposed to maximize the distance the flap can be advanced after full expansion. Zide and Karp [36] described a single or double back-cut to maximize flap advancement while allowing for donor-site closure.

Pre-expansion of a free flap donor site before microvascular free tissue transfer has added a new step to the reconstructive ladder. This technique makes possible the fabrication of flaps of a specific size and thickness [37]. Some authors have noted that the caliber of the pedicle vessels is augmented [38]. Donor sites that would otherwise be too bulky can provide tissue that is thinner as a result of the atrophy of fat from expansion. Donor-site closure is also facilitated [25]. It is questionable whether pre-expansion influences microvascular failure. Placement of the expander must be done carefully so as not to damage the donor-site vessels that will be used for subsequent microvascular tissue transfer. One study noted that dissection of the flap is more challenging because of the obliteration of tissue planes and the formation of a capsule in the flap donor site [25].

Regional considerations

Head and neck

Reconstruction of the head and neck presents a particular challenge, requiring expansion that avoids oral, visual, and airway compromise while preserving facial aesthetic units. Large congenital pigmented nevi of the head and neck can often be treated with expansion of local tissue. Bauer et al [39] reviewed their experience in 21 patients with lesions involving the forehead and scalp. They advocated medial advancement flaps for midline forehead lesions, serial advancement from the uninvolved hemiforehead in unilateral lesions, and transposition of medial tissue for supraorbital or temporal lesions not involving the hairline. Reconstruction of large lesions of the head and neck can be quite complex, because many of these lesions involve numerous anatomic structures, such as the scalp, forehead, eyelid, postauricular sulcus, and auricle (Fig. 1). Expansion of adjacent tissue cannot address the reconstructive needs of these unique structures, and the authors have found that combined-modality treatment is often required for optimal reconstruction [29]. This treatment often entails expanded flaps, full-thickness skin grafts (both expanded and nonexpanded), and serial excision. Split-thickness skin grafts, with the exception of those harvested from the scalp, provide a poor color and texture match for visible regions of the head and neck. The surgeon should address temporoparietal lesions with combined advancement and transposition flaps, choosing the reconstructive technique that best achieves proper orientation of hair follicles relative to the adjacent scalp.

Expansion has become the principal reconstructive technique for burn scars in the head and neck. Neck contractures should be addressed first, because intubation can be difficult and extrinsic pull may distort the adjacent face [40]. Many authors advocate placing tissue expanders superficial to the platysma in the neck to avoid excessively bulky flaps [41]. Another advantage of this technique is the avoidance of risk to the facial nerve, whose branches run deep to the platysma. The leading edge of unburned neck skin can be advanced by undermining to the level of the clavicle and advancing cephalad after expansion. If advancement flaps are insufficient, rotation or transposition flaps may be needed. Spence [13] described the use of pre-expanded supraclavicular transposition flaps to treat severe cervical scarring. Pre-expansion permits primary closure of the donor site in the majority of cases.

McCauley et al [14] presented their experience with burn alopecia in 102 children and proposed a classification scheme and corresponding treatment algorithm. Depending on the distribution of existing hair, multiple expansions must be undertaken with a combination of advancement and rotation flaps to restore the anterior hairline (Fig. 2). Patchy alopecia cannot be addressed adequately with expansion. Scalp expansion is ineffective in patients with greater than 50% hair loss, because significant thinning of existing hair will occur [40]. Hair-bearing skin may be transposed to the cheek to camouflage scars in men [41]. Neale et al [10] presented their experience with expansion of the lower face and anterior neck in 52 children and young adults and advised that expansion and subsequent advancement over the mandible should be performed with caution. Ectropion of the lip or lower eyelid and scar widening were among the complications. Flaps can be advanced from the level of the hyoid bone to the lip. The flap should be advanced caudally to avoid ectropion of the lip. Rotation may be preferred over advancement to take tension off the suture line in the lower face and cheeks [40]. Many authors advocate maximum expansion and advancement as the way to ensure minimal tension when insetting the flap in the cheek or lower face and avoid eyelid or lip ectropion [40,42]. Kawashima et al [42] advocate expansion of a cervicofacial flap for cheek defects because of its superior aesthetic result.

Tissue expansion has been applied to reconstruction of congenital and acquired deformities of the ear. The goal is to provide abundant thin, elastic, non–hair-bearing skin to drape over the cartilage framework of the reconstructed ear. Some authors report that expanders of specific shape and size should be

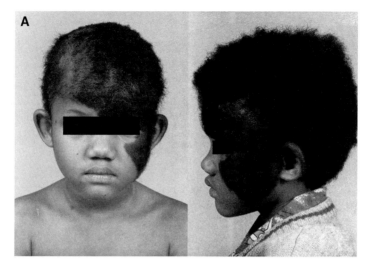

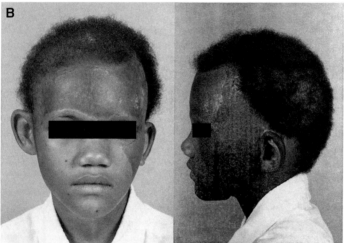

Fig. 1. (*A*) A 4-year old boy with a giant congenital pigmented nevus of the forehead, face, and scalp, involving multiple subunits. (*B*) Two years following completion of tissue expansion with flap advancement for reconstruction of the scalp and face. The forehead has been reconstructed with an expanded full thickness skin graft harvested from the abdomen.

employed [43,44]. The pocket is created away from the incision and dissected at the level of the mastoid fascia and auricular cartilage to maximize the overlying flap thickness. Caution must be exercised when expanding, because of the thin skin present here. The expander is usually removed 1 to 3 months after the final inflation, although this interval varies. At the reconstruction, capsule excision may be needed to allow the skin flap to drape over the cartilage framework, but this may compromise the blood supply to the skin [45,46]. An animal study using a porcine model disputed the importance of the capsule in providing blood to the overlying tissue [47]. Expansion of postauricular skin in acquired defects of the ear is undertaken in a similar fashion.

Expansion of scarred, contaminated, or irradiated skin may be more prone to exposure and should be undertaken with extreme caution [42].

Extremities

Expansion in the extremities has been effective in situations that preclude rotation or advancement flaps alone [48]. However, tissue expansion in these areas has limitations and is associated with a higher complication rate, particularly in the lower extremities [11,12]. Intraluminal pressure of an expander in the extremity often exceeds that placed in other regions of the body, and pressures may exceed capillary closing pressure without affecting cutaneous

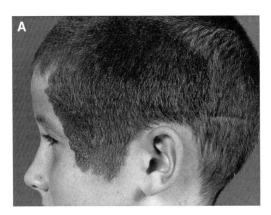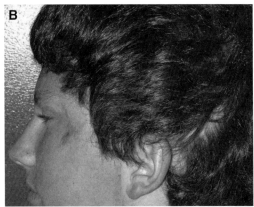

Fig. 2. (*A*) A 9-year old boy with giant congenital pigmented nevus of the left scalp and face. (*B*) Seven years following reconstruction with expanded scalp, forehead, and cheek flaps. No skin grafts were used.

capillary refill [49]. In addition, the surgeon must be aware of the potential for nerve entrapment. Expander placement and careful flap design are crucial. Patient compliance is more important here than it is in expansion of the trunk or the head and neck. For the resurfacing of large nevi, expanded full-thickness skin grafts and expanded flaps from distant regions are often used (Fig. 3) [29]. However, if the lesion can be excised in three stages or less, the authors' preference is serial excision of the lesion rather than expansion of adjacent flaps.

Trunk

Tissue expansion has been well-described for breast reconstruction and secondary burn reconstruction in adults [30,50]. The pediatric population presents unique challenges, including meningomyelocele, giant congenital nevus, and ectopia cordis. In an area with such great potential for donor tissue, expanders can exceed 1000 mL in size. Because of the abundance of donor tissue and the uniformity of the surface to be reconstructed, the authors have found the torso to be the most common location for single-modality treatment of giant congenital nevi with tissue expansion alone (Fig. 4) [29]. Ideally, the expander should have a semirigid back, especially when placed over the abdomen. The back is more difficult to expand than the abdomen or chest, necessitating longer expansion intervals. Most authors prefer to delay the second stage of expansion until the flap created for the initial advancement has firmly adhered. This delay avoids migration of the expander at the next stage.

Burn scars of the chest in a child or adolescent can be more complicated than in an adult. Both breast

development and psychological factors influence the timing of reconstruction. An area that has been treated with skin grafts or has healed by secondary intention may restrict expansion. It is recommended that expanders be placed in a submuscular position to avoid ulceration of the skin [41]. The tissue expander is subsequently replaced with a permanent implant once breast development is complete.

Complications

Tissue expansion has been associated with significant complications since its inception. Initial reports of complication rates were as high as 40% in infants and children [23]. The risks have been described in numerous studies and have been categorized by patient age, wound type, surgeon experience, and socioeconomic class. Recent series report overall complication rates in the 13% to 20% range [11,12,24]. However, the literature on complications of tissue expansion is difficult to interpret, in part because the studies are retrospective and the different authors have different definitions of "complication."

Most authors agree that minor complications do not delay the process of expansion and reconstruction, whereas major complications do. Minor complications include pain at the time of expansion, seroma, widening of scar, and temporary distortion of normal features [51]. Pain at the time of injection is related to inflation pressure. It may well be indicative of ischemia, and the injection should be stopped. If the pain goes away, inflation can continue. Dog-ears usually settle in due course. Attempts at primary correction of these should be discouraged, because flaps may be devascularized. Major complications

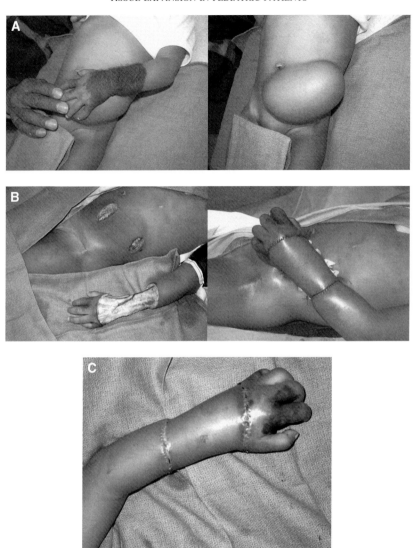

Fig. 3. (*A*) A 2-year old boy with giant congenital nevus of the left upper extremity who underwent reconstruction with tissue expansion of an abdominal flap. (*B*) After abdominal wall expansion, the nevus is excised circumferentially from the forearm and from the dorsal aspect of the wrist. The extremity is inset into the expanded abdominal flap. (*C*) The expanded abdominal flap after division of the pedicle. The patient subsequently had an expanded full-thickness skin graft harvested from the abdomen to resurface the palm and involved digits.

include hematoma, infection, expander exposure and extrusion, implant failure, and flap ischemia. Exposure may occur as a result of poor skin closure or incorrect placement of the expander [51].

Overall complications in the pediatric population by anatomic region seem to be greatest in the extremities, particularly in the lower extremities. Pisarski et al [12] reported a series of 281 expanders placed in 224 patients from 1987 to 1995 at the Shriners Burn Center in Cincinnati. These authors

found that complications were most prevalent in the lower extremity, followed by the head and neck. Another series of 180 expanders placed in 82 children demonstrated that extremity expansion resulted in more complications than did expansion in other regions, although statistical significance was questionable [11]. Elias et al [23] reported that the scalp, followed by the trunk, was the region associated with the greatest rate of tissue expander–related complications. In contrast, other series, including a large one

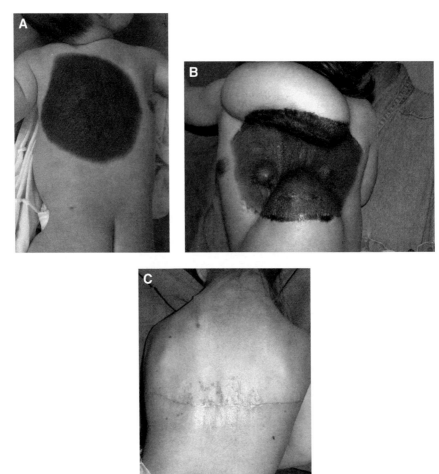

Fig. 4. (*A*) A 3-month-old girl with giant congenital pigmented nevus of the back. (*B*) At age 2 years, after placement of tissue expanders. (*C*) Two years after resection of the nevus and resurfacing with back flaps expanded in a single stage.

from Boston Children's Hospital, have found no difference in complication rates with the anatomic region treated [20,24,52].

Some debate exists over the relationship between patient age and the complication rate. In a series of 105 patients, Gibstein et al [24] found that children 1 to 12 years of age were at higher risk for developing wound disruption or expander deflation than were infants and adolescents. Another series found that children under age 7 years were at higher risk for complications [11].

Patients undergoing expansion for burn reconstruction have been considered by some to be at higher risk for complications. A series from the Shriners Burn Institute in Cincinnati reported an overall complication rate of 30% from 1984 to 1987

[33]. However, a subsequent report from the same center for 1987 to 1995 showed a rate of only 18% [12]. The authors emphasize that a "learning curve" exists—a point that is highlighted by a series from an urban hospital. The authors of that report concluded that their overall complication rate of 65% was most likely due to the inexperience of the house staff, as well as poor patient education and suboptimal follow-up [52].

Another factor that may be associated with an increased risk for complications is serial expansion [11]. However, Iconomou et al [53] found no correlation between the reason for or technique of expansion and the complication rate.

Contraindications to tissue expansion include poor patient compliance, psychiatric dysfunction, and unsuitable skin. The latter category includes unstable scars, irradiated skin, acute wounds, fresh skin grafts, and sepsis in or adjacent to the area to be expanded.

Summary

Despite its potential complications, tissue expansion in the pediatric population is an effective reconstructive modality. Because of the significant patient and family cooperation and effort needed in the expansion process, patients and families who are cooperative and compliant tend to have the best outcomes. Effective education and guidance, beginning preoperatively and continuing throughout the expansion process, are imperative. Although most of the reported complications may delay final reconstruction, few complications prevent the ultimate success of the reconstruction. For instance, expander rupture is treated by expander replacement, and expander exposure is treated by removal of the expander, advancement of the partially expanded flaps, and reinsertion of another expander once the flaps are healed. In both cases, the final reconstruction is delayed but not lost. Those surgeons who practice tissue expansion on a regular basis and are familiar with the best ways of handling complications as they arise will achieve optimal outcomes. The critical factors in achieving success are proper patient selection, thorough preoperative planning, parent and patient education, meticulous technique, and the ability to modify the reconstructive plan for each patient based on his or her clinical response.

References

[1] Neumann C. The expansion of an area of skin by progressive distention of a subcutaneous balloon. Plast Reconstr Surg 1957;19:124–30.

[2] Radovan C. Adjacent flap development using expandable silastic implant. Presented at the Annual Meeting of the American Society of Plastic and Reconstructive Surgeons. September 27–October 2, 1976, Boston, MA. 1976.

[3] Austad ED, Rose GL. A self-inflating tissue expander. Plast Reconstr Surg 1982;70:588–94.

[4] Argenta LC, Watanabe MJ, Grabb WC. The use of tissue expansion in head and neck reconstruction. Ann Plast Surg 1983;11:31–7.

[5] Johnson TM, Lowe L, Brown MD, Sullivan MJ, Nelson BR. Histology and physiology of tissue expansion. J Dermatol Surg Oncol 1993;19:1074–8.

[6] Takei T, Mills I, Katsuyuki A, et al. Molecular basis for tissue expansion: clinical implications for the surgeon. Plast Reconstr Surg 1998;101:247–58.

[7] Austad ED, Pasyk KA, McClatchey KD, Cherry GW. Histomorphologic evaluation of guinea pig skin and soft tissue after controlled tissue expansion. Plast Reconstr Surg 1982;70:704–10.

[8] Vander Kolk CA, McCann JJ, Knight KR, O'Brien B. Some further characteristics of expanded tissue. Clin Plast Surg 1987;14:447–53.

[9] Pasyk K, Argenta L, Austad ED. Histopathology of human expanded tissue. Clin Plast Surg 1987;14: 435–45.

[10] Neale HW, Kurtzmann LC, Goh KB, et al. Tissue expanders in the lower face and anterior neck in pediatric burn patients: limitations and pitfalls. Plast Reconstr Surg 1993;91:624–31.

[11] Friedman RM, Ingram AE, Rohrich RJ, et al. Risk factors for complications in pediatric tissue expansion. Plast Reconstr Surg 1996;98:1242–6.

[12] Pisarski GP, Mertens D, Warden GD, Neale HW. Tissue expander complications in the pediatric burn patient. Plast Reconstr Surg 1998;102:1008–12.

[13] Spence RJ. Experience with novel uses of tissue expanders in burn reconstruction of the face and neck. Ann Plast Surg 1992;28:453–64.

[14] McCauley RL, Oliphant JR, Robson MC. Tissue expansion in the correction of burn alopecia: classification and methods of correction. Ann Plast Surg 1990;25:103–15.

[15] Bauer BS, Vicari FA, Richard ME, Schwed R. Expanded full-thickness skin grafts in children: case selection, planning, and management. Plast Reconstr Surg 1993;92:59–69.

[16] Sawyer MG, Minde K, Zuker RM. The burned child—scarred for life? Burns 1982;9:205–13.

[17] Petres J, Muller RPA. Treatment of congenital pigmented nevi by dermabrasion. In: Happle R, Grosshans E, editors. Pediatric dermatology. Berlin: Sprigner-Verlag; 1987. p. 135.

[18] Quaba A. Reconstruction of a post-traumatic ear defect using tissue expansion: 30 years after Neumann. Plast Reconstr Surg 1988;82:521–4.

[19] Vergnes P, Taieb A, Maleville J, et al. Repeated skin expansion for excision of congenital giant nevi in infancy and childhood. Plast Reconstr Surg 1993;91: 450–5.

[20] Iconomou TG, Michelow BJ, Zuker RM. Tissue expansion in the pediatric patient. Ann Plast Surg 1993;31:134–40.

[21] Bauer BS, Vicari FA, Richard ME. The role of tissue expansion in pediatric plastic surgery. Clin Plast Surg 1990;17:101–12.

[22] Paletta C, Campbell E, Shehadi SJ. Tissue expanders in children. Clin Plast Surg 1991;28:22–5.

[23] Elias DL, Baird WL, Zubowicz VN. Applications and complications of tissue expansion in pediatric surgery. J Pediatr Surg 1991;26:15–21.

[24] Gibstein LA, Abramson DL, Bartlett RA, et al. Tissue

expansion in children: a retrospective study of complications. Ann Plast Surg 1997;38:358–64.

[25] Hallock GG. Preexpansion of free flap donor sites used in reconstruction after burn injury. J Burn Care Rehabil 1995;16:646–53.

[26] van Rappard JHA, Molenaar J, van Doorn K, et al. Surface-area increase in tissue expansion. Plast Reconstr Surg 1988;82:833–9.

[27] Duits EHA, Molenaar J, van Rappard JHA. The modeling of skin expanders. Plast Reconstr Surg 1989; 83:362–7.

[28] Wiselander JB. Tissue expansion in the head and neck. Scand J Plast Reconstr Surg Hand Surg 1991; 25:47–56.

[29] Gosain AK, Santoro TD, Larson DL, Gingrass RP. Giant congenital nevi: a 20-year experience and an algorithm for their management. Plast Reconstr Surg 2001;108:622–31.

[30] Radovan C. Tissue expansion in soft-tissue reconstruction. Plast Reconstr Surg 1984;74:482–92.

[31] Jackson IT, Sharpe DT, Polley J, et al. Use of external reservoirs in tissue expansion. Plast Reconstr Surg 1987;80:266–73.

[32] Lozano S, Drucker M. Use of tissue expanders with external ports. Ann Plast Surg 2000;44:14–7.

[33] Neale HW, High RM, Billmire DA, et al. Complications of controlled tissue expansion in the pediatric burn patient. Plast Reconstr Surg 1988;82: 840–5.

[34] Hallock G. Safety of clinical overinflation of tissue expanders. Plast Reconstr Surg 1995;96:153–7.

[35] Hallock GG. Maximum overinflation of tissue expanders. Plast Reconstr Surg 1987;80:567–9.

[36] Zide BM, Karp NS. Maximizing gain from rectangular tissue expanders. Plast Reconstr Surg 1992;90: 500–4.

[37] Russell RC, Khouri RK, Upton J, et al. The expanded scapular flap. Plast Reconstr Surg 1995;96:896–7.

[38] Iwahira Y, Maruyama Y. Expanded reduced latissimus dorsi flap. Eur J Plast Surg 1991;14:280–4.

[39] Bauer BS, Few JW, Chavez CD, et al. The role of tissue expansion in the management of large con-

[40] MacLennan SE, Corcoran JF, Neale HW. Tissue expansion in head and neck burn reconstruction. Clin Plast Surg 2000;27:121–32.

[41] Marks MW, Argenta LC, Thornton JW. Burn management: the role of tissue expansion. Clin Plast Surg 1987;14:543–50.

[42] Kawashima T, Yamada A, Ueda K, Asato H, Harii K. Tissue expansion in facial reconstruction. Plast Reconstr Surg 1994;94:944–50.

[43] Hata Y, Hosokawa K, Yano K, et al. Correction of congenital microtia using the tissue expander. Plast Reconstr Surg 1989;84:742–3.

[44] Sasaki GH. Tissue expansion in reconstruction of acquired auricular defects. Clin Plast Surg 1990;17: 327–38.

[45] Bauer BS. The role of tissue expansion in reconstruction of the ear. Clin Plast Surg 1990;17:319–25.

[46] Tanino R, Miyasaka M. Reconstruction of microtia using tissue expander. Clin Plast Surg 1990;17:339–53.

[47] Brobmann GF, Huber J. Effects of different shaped tissue expanders on transluminal pressure, oxygen tension, histopathologic changes, and skin expansion in pigs. Plast Reconstr Surg 1985;76:731–6.

[48] Borenstein A, Yaffe B, Seidmann DS, et al. Tissue expansion in reconstruction of postburn contracture of the first web space of the hand. Ann Plast Surg 1991;26:463–5.

[49] VanBeek AL, Adson MH. Tissue expansion in the upper extremity. Clin Plast Surg 1987;14:535–42.

[50] Radovan C. Breast reconstruction after mastectomy using the temporary expander. Plast Reconstr Surg 1982;69:195–208.

[51] Lari A. Tissue expansion. J R Coll Surg Edinb 1992; 37:149–54.

[52] Youm T, Margiotta M, Kasabian A, Karp N. Complications of tissue expansion in a public hospital. Ann Plast Surg 1999;42:396–402.

[53] Iconomou TG, Michelow BJ, Zuker RM. The relative risk of tissue expansion in the pediatric patient with burns. J Burn Care Rehabil 1993;14:51–4.

ELSEVIER
SAUNDERS

Clin Plastic Surg 32 (2005) 45 – 52

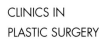
CLINICS IN
PLASTIC SURGERY

Current trends in pediatric microsurgery

Joseph M. Serletti, MD, FACS

Division of Plastic Surgery, Department of Surgery, University of Rochester Medical Center, Box 661, 601 Elmwood Avenue,
Rochester, NY 14642, USA

Free tissue transfer has become a routine method for the reconstruction of a variety of defects and is commonly employed in both the university and community hospital setting. Free tissue transfer has most often been reported in adult patients and is used to reconstruct defects caused by trauma, tumor, or vascular insufficiency. The types of tissue commonly transferred include muscle with skin, muscle with skin graft, fasciocutaneous flaps, and osteocutaneous flaps. Several series have reported on free tissue transfer specifically in children, addressing both the similarities and differences employed in the special patient population [1–3]. This article reviews common microsurgical practices used in treating pediatric patients and discusses etiologies, donor site selection issues, technical considerations including recipient site selection, and the potential for growth disturbances at both the recipient and donor sites.

Etiologies

The common etiologies for defects requiring free tissue transfer in the adult population include trauma and tumor and occasionally vascular insufficiency. The etiologies in the pediatric population include trauma and tumor as well, although there are significant differences within what is seen in trauma between adults and children and what is seen in tumor between these two groups. A frequent etiology in the pediatric population is the correction of congenital defects, which are less commonly treated in adults [1–3].

E-mail address: joseph_serletti@urmc.rochester.edu

Trauma

Trauma represents one of the most common reasons for pediatric hospital admissions [1,4]. As a result, the most common cause for a child requiring a free tissue transfer is from trauma. Vehicular trauma is one of the most common causes of this. In vehicular trauma in adults, the common injuries requiring free tissue transfer are typically open tibia fractures or severe open injuries to the ankle or foot. These types of defects are less common in children, most likely because of the plasticity of their bones as well as car seats, restraints, and children seated in the rear passenger compartment. Pedestrian injuries are more likely to result in significant soft tissue and osseus disruption of the lower extremity in children requiring free tissue reconstruction. When such injuries like open tibia fractures and open foot and ankle injuries occur in children, they are treated similar to adults [4–9].

Lawn mower injuries are one of the most common reasons for the use of free tissue transfer for trauma in children. Lawn mower injuries tend to occur in younger children with a mean age of 7. These injuries occur as a result of the patient operating the lawn mower, as a passenger on the mower, or most commonly, as an inadvertent bystander. Riding lawn mowers are associated with more severe injuries and longer hospitalizations. The injuries requiring microsurgical interventions include traumatic amputations as well as severe soft tissue injuries with exposure of joints, tendons, or bones. Because of the tendency for extensive soft tissue disruption and loss as well as wound contamination, muscle flaps are generally used for reconstructing these defects. The most common muscles used for reconstructing lawn mower

0094-1298/05/$ – see front matter © 2005 Elsevier Inc. All rights reserved.
doi:10.1016/j.cps.2004.10.002

defects include the latissimus dorsi and the rectus abdominis (Fig. 1) [10,11].

Another common traumatic etiology for free flap reconstruction in children is for burn injuries, both acute burns and late burn scar contracture [12–14]. Free tissue transfer has been employed in the management of severe full thickness burns with exposure of vital structures such as bone devoid of periosteum, tendon without paratenon, cartilage without perichondrium, or an exposed joint space. When such burn injuries occur in children, free tissue transfer is usually employed so as to provide for stable soft tissue reconstruction of these severe burn wounds. In less severe burns treated with dressing changes or skin grafting procedures, late, debilitating burn scar contracture can occur around any flexion point. These contracted burn scars can result in both substantial functional and aesthetic deformity. Commonly affected areas include the anterior neck as well as the upper and lower extremities. Free fasciocutaneous flaps have been used for the correction of these contracted burn scars. The affected area is released by division or resection of the burn scar tissues. Once fully released, an appropriately sized fasciocutaneous

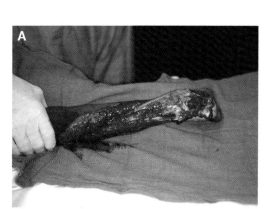
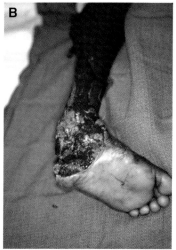
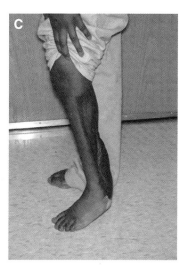
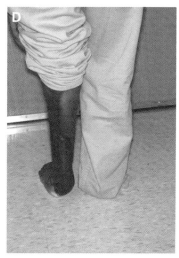

Fig. 1. (*A*) Posterior aspect of the leg and heel showing severe soft tissue loss with exposure of the calcaneous. This injury occurred in a 3-year-old girl following an injury from a riding lawn mower in which the patient was a passenger. (*B*) Medial aspect of injury showing exposure of the calcaneous. (*C*) Lateral view of leg 10 years following coverage with a free latissimus muscle and skin graft. There have been no growth disturbances in this extremity during the extended follow-up period. (*D*) Posterior aspect of healed leg and heel 10 years following injury and reconstruction.

flap is selected and used to resurface the released burn scar area. Common fasciocutaneous flaps for burn scar release include the scapular or parascapular flap, the radial forearm flap, the lateral arm flap, and the anterolateral thigh flap. Occasionally, the released surface area can exceed the dimensions of any of these flaps. In these situations, preoperative expansion of the selected fasciocutaneous flap has been used to increase the usable flap dimensions [15].

Replantation continues to represent one of the most challenging areas for success within the field of reconstructive microsurgery. Children, in particularly, are considered candidates for replantation of severed parts because of their superior recuperative abilities. For this reason, digit, hand, and major limb including lower extremity amputations are considered for replantation in children even with severe crush or avulsive injuries. Successful free tissue transfer in children mimics that seen in adults, with success rates in the range of 96% to 98%. Successful replantation has always been below the rates seen in free tissue transfer, with success rates in children in the range of 80% to 87% [16].

Congenital defects

Another area where free tissue transfer is employed in the pediatric patient population is in the treatment of congenital deformities, particularly of the head and neck region. Because of the established success of free tissue transfer in pediatric patients, earlier surgical intervention has been performed for congenital facial deformities in an effort to minimize the associated psychological trauma [17–20]. Common congenital facial abnormalities that are treated with free tissue transfer include Romberg's hemifacial atrophy, hemifacial microsomia, facial clefting, and Treacher Collins syndrome [17–22]. Most of these patients have some component of facial asymmetry with both soft tissue and osseus elements. Most free flap reconstructions for these abnormalities have used soft tissue alone for recontouring both the soft tissue and osseus defects. Osteocutaneous flaps have been used less commonly in an attempt to correct both bony and soft tissue deficiencies. Bony correction, including osteotomy, can be performed simultaneously with the free flap soft tissue augmentation. Because of the greater reliability and predictability of free flap soft tissue augmentations, free flaps are now more commonly used for the hemifacial defects compared with staged dermal fat grafts. The most common free flap for soft tissue augmentation is the scapular or parascapular flap. This flap provides for reliable thickness, can be safely contoured, avoids migration,

and matures well with facial growth and development (Fig. 2). Other choices for hemifacial augmentation include the groin flap, the omentum, and the gluteal flap. Free muscle flaps such as the latissimus dorsi and rectus abdominis have also been used, but the unpredictable degree of muscle atrophy makes achieving good results with these flaps challenging.

Free temporoparietal fascia free flaps have been used in reconstructing the external auricle in microtia patients [23]. The use of this technique is reserved for the patient presenting after multiple previous procedures with an unsatisfactory result. In such a patient, the overlying scarred soft tissue envelop will not allow appropriate projection of a cartilaginous framework. In addressing this type of patient, a new cartilage framework is designed and covered with a free temporoparietal fascia free flap harvested from the contralateral side. This allows for placement of a new framework within a new, unscarred soft tissue bed.

Cleft lip and palate are the most common congenital deformities of the head and neck. On occasion, a large palatal defect remains despite numerous staged attempts at closure. In such a patient, consideration can be given to closing a palatal or alveolar defect with free tissue transfer using soft tissue alone or soft tissue and bone such as a split metatarsal osteocutaneous flap [24,25].

Tumor

Neoplastic and malignant tumors can affect the pediatric population and, in certain circumstances, do give rise for the need for free flap reconstruction. One of the more common areas where free flap reconstruction is considered is in the surgical treatment of extremity and head and neck sarcomas. Research has demonstrated the efficacy of wide local resection with limb preservation without compromise to local control of the tumor. In some patients, this wide local resection will result in the exposure of bone, joint, bone allograft, previously irradiated tissues, or alloplastic prostheses, thus requiring free flap reconstruction for limb preservation (Fig. 3). Despite the need of these advanced reconstructive techniques for limb salvage, the long-term functional results in these reconstructed extremities has been quite good [1,26]. In many of the sarcoma resections, a specific muscle compartment or compartments are resected, leaving both a soft tissue deficit requiring reconstruction and a significant functional deficit in the affected extremity. In these special situations, consideration is given to providing a functional reconstruction. This is done by tagging the motor nerve or nerves to the resected muscle compartment. An appropriately sized donor

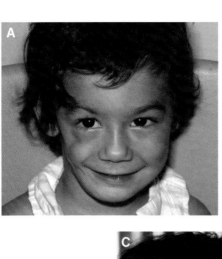
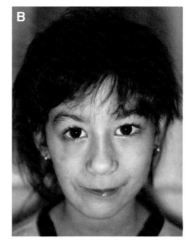
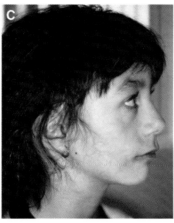

Fig. 2. (*A*) A 4-year-old girl with right-sided Romberg's hemifacial atrophy. (*B*) Anterior view of the patient 2 years following facial augmentation with a buried scapular flap. (*C*) Lateral view following a buried scapular flap for right-sided hemifacial atrophy.

muscle, usually the latissimus or gracilis, is harvested with its motor nerve and blood supply. The donor muscle is anastomosed to recipient vessels near the site of the compartment defect, and the motor nerve of the donor muscle is anastomosed to the previously tagged motor nerve from the resected compartment. The donor muscle is placed under appropriate tension and securely fixed to the proximal and distal functional ends of the resected compartment. In this way, the donor muscle serves a dual purpose. It provides for soft tissue reconstruction for limb preservation and helps to restore the functional loss of the resected compartment. Sarcoma resection can also result in a segmental bony defect. The use of the free fibular flap with or without an attached skin paddle or muscle has been helpful in reconstructing these osseus defects. The free fibular flap can be used as a single

means of providing reconstruction in small segmental defects. This can be done with a single segment of fibula or because of the segmental blood supply to fibula, the fibula can be folded on itself to provide a "double barrel" segment of bone. For larger defects, bone allograft or alloplastic prostheses are used, but here the free fibula can be of help at the junctions between the allograft and the native bone to provide for more secure consolidation at the union site.

Donor site selection

The types of tissues typically transferred in routine free flap surgery include muscle, muscle with attached skin (myocutaneous), skin and fascia (fasciocutaneous), bone, bone with attached skin (osteo-

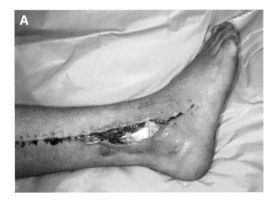
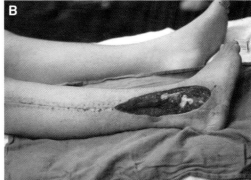
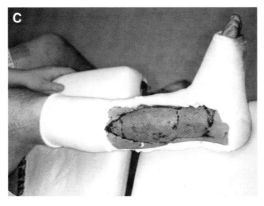

Fig. 3. (*A*) Open wound following elective resection of a synovial cell sarcoma in a 15-year-old male with exposure of the ankle joint and stabilizing hardware. (*B*) Following serial debridement, the wound is clean but the ankle joint remains exposed. (*C*) Early postoperative view following a free rectus abdominis muscle flap and skin graft for ankle joint coverage and limb preservation.

cutaneous), or bone with attached skin and muscle (oseteomyocutaneous). Either a muscle with a skin graft, a myocutaneous flap, or a fasciocutaneous flap can be selected for satisfactory reconstruction of a given defect. How do we select the best option for a particular defect, and are decisions here different because of the special age of this patient population? There are five general parameters thar direct the selection of appropriate donor tissues: wound characteristics, the length of the flap required, patient position during the surgery, contour issues, and functional and aesthetic considerations.

Wounds can be characterized as either clean or contaminated. Almost all traumatic wounds are contaminated, whereas surgically created wounds, like in elective sarcoma surgery, would be clean. Because of the better blood supply within muscle, muscle flaps are usually selected over fasciocutaneous flaps when the defect site is considered contaminated. It is felt that the muscle will perform better in that setting in terms of avoiding wound infection and achieving

satisfactory healing between the free flap tissues and the wound defect. If a particular wound has irregular geometry, multiply connected cavities, or has had previous irradiation, a muscle flap is selected over a skin flap because of the muscle's better ability to fill the dead space in such a wound.

The length of the flap is a very important selection criteria since the flap must extend from the site of the closest usable recipient vessels to the end of the defect to be reconstructed. Errors in flap length selection will require preparation of a different recipient site or the use of vein grafts, both of which makes this type of surgery even more complex and time-consuming. When length is a significant issue for reconstruction, the omentum can provide long length in adults but may not be as well developed in children. For significant length requirements in children, the latissimus dorsi muscle is usually selected.

In virtually all free flap reconstructions, surgical preparation must occur at both a recipient site and a donor site, thus allowing for the potential for two-team surgery. Simultaneous surgery at the recipient and donor sites results in shortened operative times; this is important, because any free flap surgery tends to be a lengthy procedure. When there are a variety of options for donor tissue selection, a donor tissue is selected that allows for a patient to be positioned, which will allow a two-team simultaneous surgical approach. For patients in a supine position, the rectus abdominis and the anterolateral thigh flap are examples of common choices. For patients in a decubitus or prone position, the latissimus is a common choice.

Many muscle flaps, particularly around the lower extremity, remain permanently bulky despite some muscle atrophy and represent significant long-term

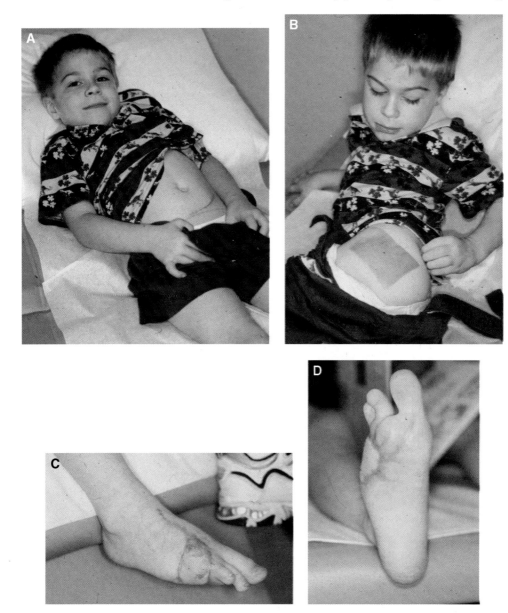

Fig. 4. (*A*) Postoperative view of a healed Pfannenstiel scar used for harvest of a limited portion of the left rectus abdominis muscle for coverage of a lawn mower injury to the foot. (*B*) The split thickness skin graft donor site is limited to the buttock and can be easily hidden with clothing, including a bathing suit. (*C*) Postoperative view of the dorsal aspect of the foot following reconstruction of an open amputation site of the lateral two toes with a free rectus abdominis and unmeshed split thickness skin graft. (*D*) Plantar view of the foot showing good contour and no breakdown on the weight-bearing surface of the reconstruction.

contour abnormalities. These contour abnormalities, particularly around the foot and ankle region, are problematic in terms of normal foot wear and athletic activities. When a defect occurs in one these contour sensitive areas, and there are no other significant flap parameters required, preference is given to a fasciocutaneous flap because of the improved final contour results achieved with these types of flaps.

Finally, the aesthetic impact of free flap reconstructions at both the recipient site and donor site cannot be underestimated in this special group of patients. In making final selections for the choice of the donor tissue transferred, much attention is given to aesthetic considerations. For example, when a muscle flap is required, preference is given to the rectus abdominis which can be harvested through a Pfannenstiel incision compared with the latissimus. A Pfannenstiel scar can be hidden with most types of clothing, including a bathing suit, whereas a latissimus scar cannot. When a skin graft is required for coverage of a muscle flap, the split thickness skin graft is harvested from the buttock, not the thigh. The skin graft is usually placed unmeshed on the muscle for better final aesthetics (Fig. 4). Endoscopic harvest approaches for a variety of flaps also play a significant potential role in flap harvest in children. Long-term functional considerations are also employed in flap selection and flap harvest. If the rectus abdominis muscle is selected, the muscle is usually split and a portion of the muscle is harvested while preserving as many functional motor nerves to the remaining rectus abdominis muscle. The latissimus can also be split so as to preserve a significant portion of functional muscle.

Technical considerations

The anatomy and soft tissue characteristics of the pediatric patient population is quite diverse, and this diversity is primarily age-related. Most pediatric patient populations are defined as newborn through 18 years of age. As they grow older, patients accumulate more and more adult soft tissue and vessel characteristics, particulary from ages 12 through 18. This age group does not usually require any special technical considerations compared with the adult population. Younger children—those ages 2 through 10—have smaller vessels and morphologic differences in their vessel walls that should be recognized by surgeons performing free flaps in this age group. An operating microscope, appropriately fine microsurgical instruments, and 10-O and 11-O microsuture

should be available. In the extremities of older children and adults, the venae comitantes of the donor artery are usually used, because the donor vein and superficial veins should be avoided. In younger children, the venae comitantes are usually too small or underdeveloped to allow for reliable venous outflow. In younger patients requiring extremity reconstruction, a superficial vein (eg, the saphenous vein) is selected because of its larger size and better match with the typical donor vein.

Growth issues

It is important to remember that for most of the pediatric patients treated with free tissue transfer, they are going to continue to grow including at or around the recipient and donor sites. There does not appear to be one or a group of transferred free flap tissues that grows more reliably than others, nor are there tissues that significantly produce growth disturbances. Most growth issues in these patients occur as a result of traumatic wounds, particularly those involving growing bone. The growth disturbances in these settings is usually not the free flap tissues but rather the underlying bone and its impaired growth from injury [27,28]. Particularly for trauma and tumor patients, a commitment to appropriate postoperative physical therapy and a return to the fullest functional activities possible seem to ensure the absence of significant growth-related issues.

Summary

Reconstructive microsurgery and free tissue transfer are commonly employed techniques in the modern-day treatment of a broad range of defects. Although most of these defects occur in the adult population, these advanced reconstructive techniques can also be affectively used in the pediatric population. Defects in children that arise from trauma, congental processes, and tumor surgery can all favorably be reconstructed with free tissue transfer. Donor tissue selection in children should give strong consideration to aesthetics and functional issues in addition to the usual parameters. Because of the smaller size of these patients and their anatomic structures, special equipment is required to reliably perform free tissue transfer. Free tissue transfer in children allows for very satisfactory functional and aesthetic results for the broad spectrum of defects reconstructed and this generally occurs without significant growth disturbances.

References

[1] Serletti JM, Schingo VA, Deuber MA, et al. Free tissue transfer in pediatric patients. Ann Plast Surg 1996;36: 561–8.

[2] Furnas DW, Turpin IM, Bernstein JM. Free flaps in young and old patients. Clin Plast Surg 1983;10: 149–54.

[3] Yucel A, Aydin Y, Yazar S, et al. Elective free-tissue transfer in pediatric patients. J Reconstr Microsurg 2001;17:27–36.

[4] Hallock GG. Efficacy of free flaps for pediatric trauma patients in an adult trauma center. J Reconstr Microsurg 1995;11:169–74.

[5] Banic A, Wulff K. Latissumus dorsi free flaps for total repair of extensive lower leg injuries in children. Plast Reconstr Surg 1987;79:769–75.

[6] Hope PG, Cole WG. Open fractures of the tibia in children. J Bone Joint Surg Br 1992;74:546–53.

[7] Skoll PJ, Hudson DA. Combined pedicled flaps for grade IIIB tibial fractures in children: a report of two patients. Ann Plast Surg 2000;44:422–5.

[8] Hahn SB, Lee JW, Jeong JH. Tendon transfer with a microvascular free flap for injured feet in children. J Bone Joint Surg Br 1998;80:86–90.

[9] Iwaya T, Harii K, Yamada A. Microvascular free flaps for the treatment of avulsion injuries of the feet in children. J Trauma 1982;22:15–9.

[10] Horowitz JH, Nichter LS, Kenney JG, et al. Lawn-mower injuries in children: lower extremity reconstruction. J Trauma 1985;25:1138–46.

[11] Loder RT, Brown KL, Zaleske DJ, et al. Extremity lawn-mower injuries in children: report by the Research Committee of the Pediatric Orthopaedic Society of North America. J Pediatr Orthop 1997;17: 360–9.

[12] DeLorenzi F, van der Hulst R, Boeckx W. Free flaps in burn reconstruction. Burns 2001;27:603–12.

[13] Mast BA, Newton ED. Aggressive use of free flaps in children for burn scar contractures and other soft-tissue deficits. Ann Plast Surg 1996;36:569–75.

[14] Shen TY, Sun YH, Cao DX, et al. The use of free flaps in burn patients: experiences with 70 flaps in 65 patients. Plast Reconstr Surg 1998;81:352–7.

[15] Cooper RL, Brown D. Pretransfer tissue expansion of a scalp free flap for burn alopecia reconstruction in a child: a case report. J Reconstruc Microsurg 1990;6: 339–43.

[16] Beris AE, Soucacos PN, Malizos KN. Microsurgery in children. Clin Orthop 1995;112–21.

[17] Siebert JW, Anson G, Longaker MT. Microsurgical correction of facial asymmetry in 60 consecutive cases. Plast Reconstr Surg 1996;97:354–63.

[18] Longaker MT, Siebert JW. Microsurgical correction of facial contour in congenital craniofacial malformations: the marriage of hard and soft tissue. Plast Reconstr Surg 1996;98:942–50.

[19] Fisher J, Jackson IT. Microvascular surgery as an adjunct to craniomaxillofacial reconstruction. Br J Plast Surg 1989;42:146–54.

[20] Hemmer KM, Marsh JL, Clement RW. Pediatric facial free flaps. J Reconstr Microsurg 1987;3:221–9.

[21] La Rossa D, Whitaker L, Dabb R, et al. The use of microvascular free flaps for soft tissue augmentation of the face in children with hemifacial microsomia. Cleft Palate J 1980;17:138–43.

[22] Inigo F, Jimenez-Murat Y, Arroyo O, et al. Restoration of facial contour in Romberg's disease and hemifacial microsomia: experience with 118 cases. Microsurgery 2000;20:167–72.

[23] Brent B, Byrd HS. Secondary ear reconstruction with cartilage grafts covered by axial, random, and free flaps of temporoparietal fascia. Plast Reconstr Surg 1983;72:141–52.

[24] Moghari Λ, Macleod ZR, Mohebbi H, et al. The use of split metatarsal osteocutaneous free flaps in palatal and alveolar defects. J Reconstr Microsurg 1989;5:307–10 [discussion: 311–2].

[25] Futran ND, Haller JR. Considerations for free-flap reconstruction of the hard palate. Arch Otolaryngol Head Neck Surg 1999;125:665–9.

[26] Serletti JM, Carras AJ, O'Keefe R, et al. Functional outcome after soft-tissue reconstruction for limb salvage after sarcoma surgery. Plast Reconstr Surg 1998; 102:1576–83 [discussion: 1584–5].

[27] Potparic Z, Rajacic N. Long-term results of weight-bearing foot reconstruction with non-innervated and and reinnervated free flaps. Br J Plast Surg 1997;50: 176–81.

[28] Harris PG, Letrosne E, Caouette-Laberge L, et al. Long-term follow-up of coverage of weight bearing surface of the foot with free muscular flap in a pediatric population. Microsurgery 1994;15:424–9.

ELSEVIER
SAUNDERS

Clin Plastic Surg 32 (2005) 53 – 64

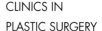

CLINICS IN
PLASTIC SURGERY

Deformational plagiocephaly: diagnosis, prevention, and treatment

Joseph E. Losee, MD, FACS, FAAP[a,b,]*, A. Corde Mason, MD, FAAP[a]

[a]*Department of Surgery, University of Pittsburgh Medical School, 3550 Terrace Street, Pittsburgh, PA 15261, USA*
[b]*Pediatric Plastic Surgery, Children's Hospital of Pittsburgh, 3705 Fifth Avenue, Pittsburgh, PA 15213, USA*

The term plagiocephaly, derived from the Greek words *plagio* (oblique, twisted, or slant) and *kephale* (head), describes an asymmetric cranium. Cranial asymmetry has multiple origins. In utero, asymmetry may develop secondary to genetic abnormalities that permit early sutural synostosis, distorting the developing neurocranium early in gestation. Such is the case in several recognized syndromes of craniosynostosis. Additionally, mechanical forces exerted on the fetal skull due to multiple gestations, reduced maternal pelvic volume, or fetal neurologic abnormalities may lead to a misshapen, asymmetric skull. Ex utero, the neonatal cranium is recognized to be quite malleable, and persistent mechanical forces acting on it can lead to a desired or undesired molding effect.

Historically, the growing skull's pliability was recognized by cultures worldwide [1]. The Peruvian custom of head molding was so prevalent that very few recovered skulls do not show evidence of molding. It is believed that Peruvians viewed people with long, broad heads as healthier and stronger. People in various societies have practiced intentional skull molding to set themselves or their families apart from the masses. Distinctive head shape often designated nobility, as in the case of the Egyptian queen Nefertiti and her daughters.

Various cultures have shaped infant heads using external compression to inhibit growth in one direction, while permitting compensatory growth in another. This method capitalizes on the unique engineering and architecture of the newborn skull. Composed of multiple suture-segregated bones, the skull must accommodate the external forces presented to it while negotiating the birth canal. To this end, the skull bones must shift in position and override one another to permit successful passage. Post partum, the bones of the "molded" infant skull typically resettle into a symmetric form and ultimately close, resulting in the accepted uniform head shape. This process is predicated on underlying brain growth. Placement of fixed external devices on newborns' heads can modify this resettling and shape the head into a desired contour.

Plagiocephaly: classification

As already noted, the contour of the head of vaginally delivered healthy newborns is frequently misshapen. However, asymmetry at birth that does not rapidly and spontaneously resolve, or asymmetry that evolves in the first several postnatal months, should prompt concern. Cranial asymmetry has a convoluted history within the craniofacial literature and can prompt confusion because of inconsistent nomenclature and misdiagnosis. For diagnosis and treatment, plagiocephaly should initially be categorized as either anterior or posterior. Subsequently, it can be classified as synostotic or nonsynostotic plagiocephaly [2]. Typically, anterior synostotic plagiocephaly results from unicoronal craniosynostosis, whereas anterior nonsynostotic plagiocephaly is rare and results from external forces acting on the

* Corresponding author. Pediatric Plastic Surgery, Children's Hospital of Pittsburgh, 3705 Fifth Avenue, Pittsburgh, PA 15213.

E-mail address: joseph.losee@chp.edu (J.E. Losee).

0094-1298/05/$ – see front matter © 2005 Elsevier Inc. All rights reserved.
doi:10.1016/j.cps.2004.08.003

neonatal skull. Posterior synostotic plagiocephaly results from lambdoid craniosynostosis, which is very rare, whereas posterior nonsynostotic plagiocephaly results from external forces and is quite prevalent today. Various names have been assigned to posterior nonsynostotic plagiocephaly, including posterior plagiocephaly, postural plagiocephaly, occipital plagiocephaly, and deformational plagiocephaly. Over the past decade, confusion over the etiology, diagnosis, and treatment of posterior plagiocephaly has resulted in the misdiagnosis and unnecessary surgical treatment of children with nonsynostotic plagiocephaly. For the purposes of this article, the authors refer to posterior nonsynostotic plagiocephaly as deformational plagiocephaly.

Isolated posterior synostotic plagiocephaly, or lambdoid craniosynostosis, is a rare form of craniosynostosis and has an incidence of 0.003% to 5% [3–5]. Infants with lambdoid craniosynostosis are noted to have occipital flattening at the time of birth. The cause of craniosynostosis is not fully understood. Familial patterns suggest that there may be pedigrees in which the disorder is inherited. Some researchers believe that intrauterine mechanical forces exerted on the developing neurocranium play a notable role. One study reported that infants with lambdoid craniosynostosis had a nearly threefold increase in the length of the first stage of labor. The authors hypothesized that sustained mechanical compressive forces within the birth canal between the fetal head and the maternal pelvis played a role in the development of plagiocephaly in these infants [6]. Preterm labor was also found to occur with greater frequency in those infants affected. Additionally, it has been suggested that sex differences in head growth and size predispose the male fetal head to the development of craniosynostosis. Typically greater in size, the male cranium is more likely to be affected by the intrauterine forces exerted on vaginal delivery, resulting in the greater male than female incidence of craniosynostosis. How these forces exerted on the third-trimester neurocranium translate into early craniosynostosis is not understood. Currently, suture pathology at the molecular pathway level is being elucidated [7].

Deformational plagiocephaly

Deformational plagiocephaly is occipital flattening that presents in the perinatal period as a unilateral or bilateral deformity and is often associated with changes to the anterior craniofacial skeleton. It is the most common type of plagiocephaly, with a prevalence ranging from 5% to 48% of healthy newborns

[3]. Though deformational plagiocephaly is not a new phenomenon, its recognition and diagnosis have become more common since the early 1990s, when the American Academy of Pediatrics (AAP) made its recommendation to place newborns to sleep in a supine position. This practice guideline has had impressive effects on the incidence of sudden infant death, reducing it from 40% to 9%. Compliance with the recommendation, however, has resulted in an estimated 51% of infants spending most of the time on their backs [8,9]. Accordingly, the infant skull generally comes to rest on one side of the occiput, and a persistent sleep position develops. This persistent sleep pattern leads to sustained forces upon the developing and malleable infant skull. Early evidence of these pressures may be localized occipital alopecia. If they are allowed to continue, abnormal molding or flattening of the underlying cranium occurs, resulting in deformational plagiocephaly.

Several studies have looked at the demographics of deformational plagiocephaly. A male predominance has been consistently observed, with a distribution ranging from 60% to 70% [10–12]. A further predilection for laterality has been demonstrated, with the majority of cases right-sided unilateral (57%–70% right-sided, 24%–30% left-sided, 4%–18% bilateral) [10,13,14]. Because the AAP "Back to Sleep" campaign has been embraced most readily by white populations, it is not surprising to find an increased incidence of deformational plagiocephaly among white children (95% white, 2% African American, 2% Hispanic) [9,10,15]. Further investigation has revealed a significant incidence of multiparity among the deformational plagiocephaly population, with an incidence of twinning ranging from 8% to 12.4% [10,11,16–18]. The association of prematurity with deformational plagiocephaly has been inconsistent, with some authors reporting no increased incidence and others an incidence as high as 18.6% [10,11,16,17]. The significant associated finding of contralateral torticollis is very prevalent, with an incidence of 3% to 20% [10,12,16].

Classically, deformational plagiocephaly is a postnatal acquired condition. However, it is important to recognize that a condition of congenital deformational plagiocephaly has been found to occur up to 10% of the time [10]. Congenital deformational plagiocephaly is thought to be secondary to intrauterine compression between the pelvic brim and lumbosacral spine and persistent right occiput transverse lie. Acquired deformational plagiocephaly is thought to occur when infants are placed supine and assume a "position of comfort" that most likely corresponds to their previous intrauterine lie. Newborns are typically unable to lift and midline their heads until 3 months of life, when neuromotor control has matured. When the infant is allowed to develop a persistent sleep position, this behavior is subsequently difficult or impossible to change. The persistent sleep position, generally with the head turned to the right, results in constant compressive forces exerted against the expanding infant skull. These forces result in a unilateral occipital flattening and secondary anterior displacement of the ipsilateral craniofacial features, including the ear, forehead, and cheek. Furthermore, the infant's ability to roll independently from the supine to prone position is not acquired until 5 or 6 months of life. By the time the infant reaches this developmental milestone, the "position of comfort" and established sleep pattern preclude self-correction.

Diagnosis

Distinguishing between synostotic and nonsynostotic posterior plagiocephaly has proved to be challenging. The unanticipated effects of supine sleep positioning led to a marked increase in the number of infants presenting with occipital plagiocephaly in the 1990s. Many of these infants were mistakenly diagnosed as having lambdoid craniosynostosis, resulting in a perceived inexplicable epidemic in some centers [4,19–21]. Our current understanding, largely based on the work of the Seattle Craniofacial Center, makes possible effective discrimination between these two conditions on the basis of a careful history and attentive examination [4,22].

Although infants with lambdoid craniosynostosis and deformational plagiocephaly both have occipital flattening, the time of first recognition tends to differ. Infants with lambdoid craniosynostosis have recognized asymmetry at birth, which may progress as the infant grows postnatally. This presentation differs from that of the typical infant with acquired deformational plagiocephaly, who has a normal and symmetric head at birth yet develops an asymmetry over subsequent weeks or months.

Examination, therefore, is the key to the diagnosis. The infant should be observed from anterior, posterior, and vertex positions. Initially, the infant is placed in the parental lap facing forward, and the examiner evaluates the anterior craniofacial skeleton for symmetry. In this view, head tilt and twist, as well as the forehead, orbits, midface, and mandible, are critically assessed. In up to 80% of infants with typical unilateral deformational plagiocephaly, the ipsilateral forehead is displaced anteriorly, creating the illusion of asymmetric enlargement [14]. The

ipsilateral palpebral fissure is often vertically elongated, creating the illusion of an overly "open" eye. The senior author has seen several children referred with concern over orbital tumors, when, in fact, the underlying condition of ipsilateral deformational plagiocephaly had resulted in the illusion of ipsilateral proptosis. The ipsilateral cheek is also often displaced anteriorly, again creating the illusion of asymmetric enlargement (Fig. 1). Likewise, the senior author has evaluated several children referred with the potential diagnosis of hemifacial microsomia, when, in fact, the underlying contralateral deformational plagiocephaly had displaced the ipsilateral face anteriorly, resulting in the appearance of asymmetric enlargement on the affected side of the face and of hemifacial microsomia on the unaffected side. The mandibular midline can be displaced to the affected side, a result of contralateral head tilt and ipsilateral head twist due to associated torticollis. In severe cases, the occlusion may even be affected, with an upward cant on the affected side.

The infant is then turned facing the parent as the examiner evaluates the posterior head. Careful attention is directed to the mastoid skull. In typical deformational plagiocephaly, the mastoid skull base is symmetric (Fig. 2). In lambdoid craniosynostosis, an expected compensatory growth results in bulging of the ipsilateral mastoid skull base and contralateral parietal eminence (Fig. 3). The affected suture in lambdoid craniosynostosis will have a palpable external ridging. The infant is next placed "face supine," with the head in the examiner's lap and feet in the parent's lap, for the vertex perspective. In typical deformational plagiocephaly, an occipital flatness is

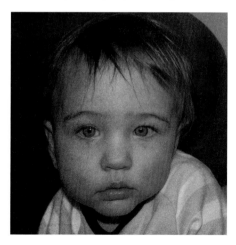

Fig. 1. Anterior view of a child with right-sided posterior plagiocephaly demonstrates anterior craniofacial changes: an advanced forehead, ear, and cheek.

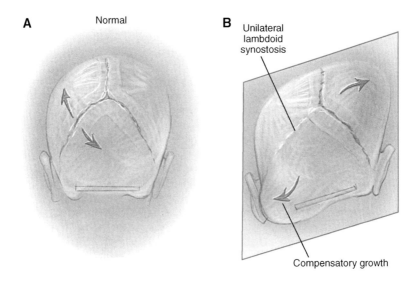

Fig. 2. Differences between synostotic and nonsynostotic posterior plagiocephaly, posterior view. Solid arrows indicate growth vectors; clear mark indicates skull base axis. (*A*) Posterior deformational plagiocephaly, skull base horizontal, no mastoid bulging. (*B*) Lambdoid craniosynostosis, ipsilateral compensatory mastoid bossing, and contralateral parietal compensatory bossing. (*From* Lin KY, Ogle RC, Jane JA, editors. Craniofacial surgery: science and surgical technique. Philadelphia: WB Saunders; 2002. p. 241; with permission.)

associated with ipsilateral ear, forehead, and cheek anterior displacement, resulting in the characteristic parallelogram skull shape (Figs. 4 and 5). In lambdoid craniosynostosis, a lack of anterior displacement of the ipsilateral forehead results in a trapezoidal skull shape (Table 1).

As noted earlier, associated contralateral muscular torticollis is frequently seen in children with deforma-

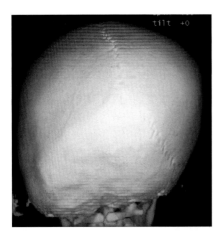

Fig. 3. CT scan, posterior view, left-sided lambdoid craniosynostosis. Note obliterated suture with ectocranial ridge, ipsilateral mastoid bulging, and contralateral parietal eminence bulging.

tional plagiocephaly. In the anterior view, particular attention is paid to head tilt and twist. Infants with deformational plagiocephaly, both acquired and congenital, routinely have contralateral sternocleidomastoid (SCM) muscle "stiffness" rather than true muscle atrophy and fibrosis. This condition is probably due to persistent intrauterine or postnatal positioning and a lack of normal range of motion. The normal SCM muscle functions in tilting the head ipsilaterally and twisting it contralaterally. In typical deformational plagiocephaly, the contralateral SCM muscle is "stiff" and foreshortened, resisting full extension. This "stiffness" results in a contralateral head tilt and ipsilateral head twist (Fig. 6). With the child's head in the examiner's lap, palpation of the contralateral SCM often demonstrates a slight tightness and tenderness. Attempts at contralateral head twist are met with resistance and agitation on the part of the patient, confirming the diagnosis of muscular torticollis.

Radiographic evaluation is rarely indicated and usually serves to complement the history and physical examination, or as a preoperative tool when lambdoid craniosynostosis is suspected. Plain radiographs of the skull may be used when the clinical examination is equivocal; however, they are best used to confirm sutural patency, ruling out craniosynostosis. When craniosynostosis is suspected, a high-resolution, three-dimensional CT scan of the head is obtained.

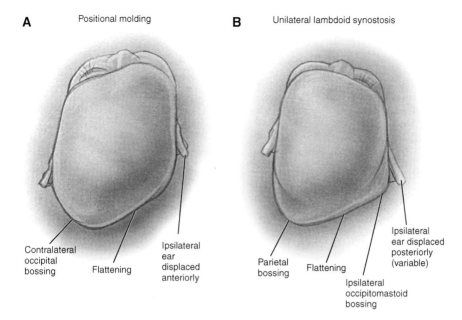

Fig. 4. Vertex view of (*A*) right-sided deformational plagiocephaly and (*B*) right-sided lamboid craniosynostosis with summary of some differences. (*From* Lin KY, Ogle RC, Jane JA, editors. Craniofacial surgery: science and surgical technique. Philadelphia: WB Saunders; 2002. p. 242; with permission.)

This study will assess brain morphology, characterize skull-base anomalies, and define cranial contour.

Losee et al [23] recently defined the radiographic diagnosis of deformational plagiocephaly. Lambdoid sutures in patients with deformational plagiocephaly have areas of focal fusion, endocranial ridging, narrowing, sclerosis, and perisutural thinning, and all

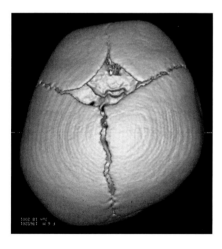

Fig. 5. CT scan, vertex view, right-sided posterior deformational plagiocephaly. Note ipsilateral occipital flattening and ipsilateral forehead anterior displacement, resulting in parallelogram-shaped head.

cases exhibit a change in orientation from overlapping to end-to-end (Fig. 7). These sutural changes historically have been erroneously attributed to lambdoid craniosynostosis, which contributed to the falsely elevated incidence of lambdoid craniosynostosis in the early 1990s. In contrast, the lambdoid sutures in craniosynostosis routinely demonstrate complete obliteration, as well as ectocranial and endocranial ridging, and are associated with a pattern of ipsilateral mastoid bossing and contralateral parietal eminence bossing. Contrary to previous reports, lambdoid craniosynostosis is not unique among suture fusions and presents with suture obliteration and compensatory bossing similar to other forms of craniosynostosis.

The diagnosis and treatment of children with deformational plagiocephaly are facilitated by a recently developed severity-assessment rating system [24]. This standardized rating system uses various physical findings as a means of classifying the degree of deformity. In addition, it is useful in tracking the progress made during treatment (Fig. 8).

Sequelae

Currently, controversy reigns on the question of whether deformational plagiocephaly has any poten-

Table 1
Distinguishing features between lambdoidal craniosynostosis and deformational plagiocephaly

Characteristic	Lambdoidal craniosynostosis	Deformational plagiocephaly
Vertex head shape	Trapezoid	Parallelogram
Anterior forehead displacement	Normal	Ipsilateral
Anterior facial asymmetry	May be affected	Often affected
Anterior ear displacement	None	Ipsilateral
Ipsilateral mastoid bossing	Present	Absent
Contralateral parietal bossing	Present	Absent
Suture	Palpable ridge	No palpable finding
Torticollis	Infrequent	Frequent

tial physiologic sequelae. Some authors have warned of long-lasting craniofacial changes affecting jaw function and occlusal relationships, visual disturbances, neurologic developments, and the like. However, few data exist to support these claims.

Conflicting data on the ocular sequelae of deformational plagiocephaly have been reported. Recent work by Francel and Panchal [25] has shown a detectable incidence of visual-field constriction in patients with deformational plagiocephaly, and the authors conclude that children with this disorder may have a delayed progression of visual-field development. However, Gupta et al [26] evaluated strabismus and astigmatism in 111 patients with deformational plagiocephaly and found the prevalence of both conditions in that cohort to be similar to that in the general population.

Auditory processing has been reported to be affected in children with deformational plagiocephaly. Balan et al [5] reported that infants with both synostotic and nonsynostotic plagiocephaly exhibited dramatically smaller response amplitudes to auditory event-related potentials than did controls, a result consistent with compromised brain function. Although spontaneous recovery may occur in early childhood, the authors suggested that these infants were at high risk for developmental difficulties and recommended close observation.

The potential neurodevelopmental sequelae of synostotic plagiocephaly and, more recently, of deformational plagiocephaly are being recognized. The specific effects of a fused suture on the underlying cortex and subsequent effects on neurodevelopmental pathways are unknown; however, there does appear to be an anatomic blunting of the cortex in patients with craniosynostosis. Studies have long identified an increased number of children with minor learning

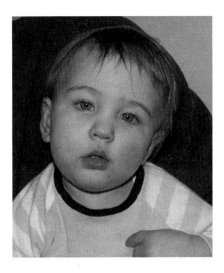

Fig. 6. Anterior view of child with right-sided posterior deformational plagiocephaly and left-sided torticollis. Note typical contralateral head tilt and ipsilateral head twist consistent with contralateral SCM muscle involvement.

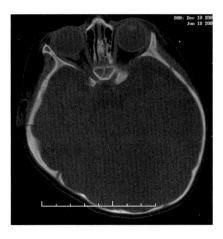

Fig. 7. Axial CT scan of right-sided deformational plagiocephaly with suture demonstrating endocranial ridging, narrowing, sclerosis, perisutural thinning, and a change in orientation from overlapping to end-to-end.

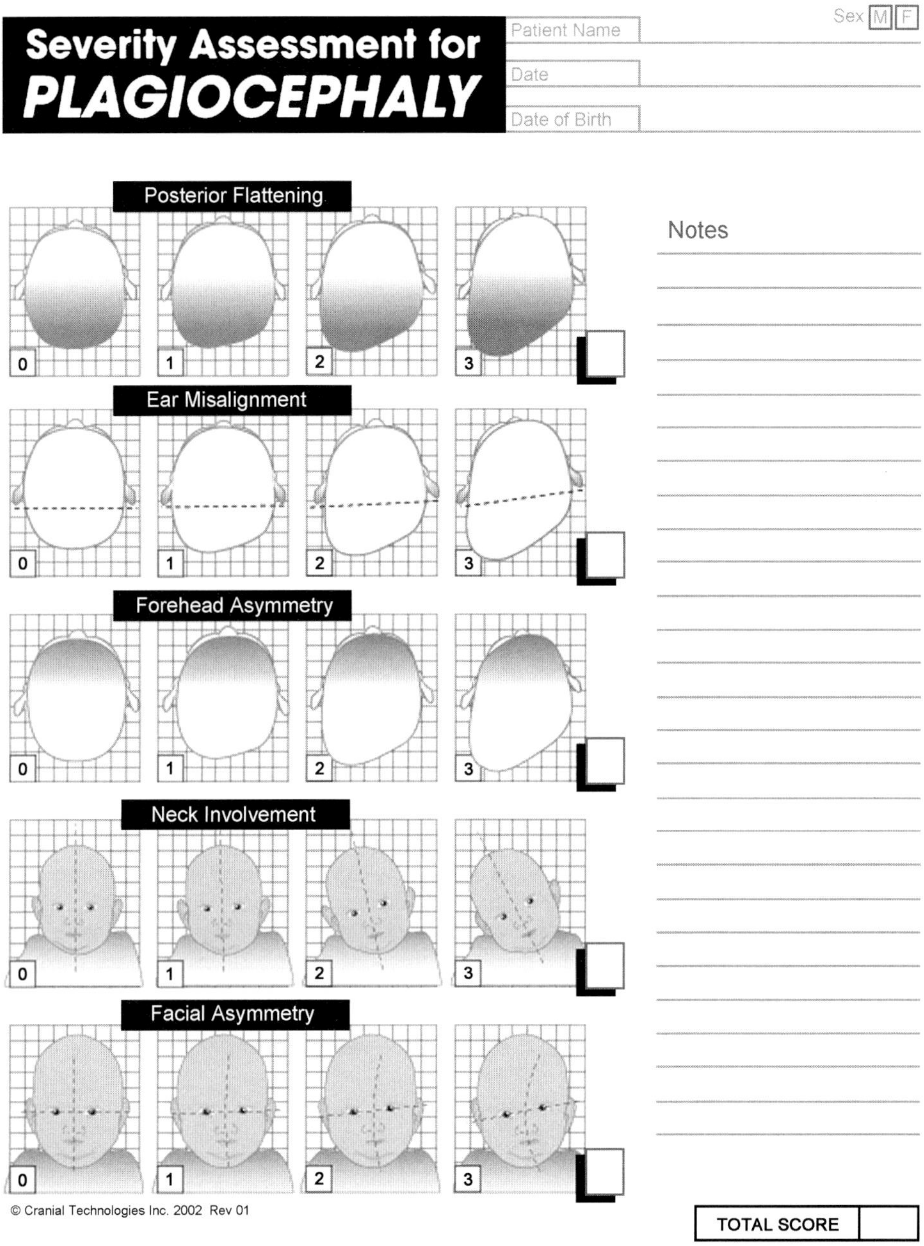

Fig. 8. Severity assessment form for plagiocephaly. (Courtesy of Cranial Technologies, Tempe, AZ, 2002; with permission.)

disorders who have single-suture craniosynostosis [27,28], and Panchal et al [29] found a significant incidence of cognitive and psychomotor developmental delays in infants with deformational plagiocephaly. Children in Panchal's study showed delays as early as 12 months that correlated with developmental delays at 4.5 years of age, suggesting that delays in the first year of life were predictive of delays in later childhood [29]. These data correlate with the findings of Miller and Clarren [30], who documented the need for special education in 40% of patients with deformational plagiocephaly in contrast to their nonaffected siblings. By school age, the authors found an increase in the number of patients with language disorders, learning disabilities, and attention deficits.

Treatment

Treatment strategies begin with prevention. Primary care providers for newborns are instrumental in educating new parents about methods of reducing the risk of deformational plagiocephaly. Supine sleep position has significantly reduced the incidence of sudden infant deaths, and it should be stressed during unattended sleep periods. However, a considerable amount of prone positioning or "tummy time" for the awake, observed infant is recommended. This measure both prevents the evolution of a persistent sleep pattern and promotes shoulder-girdle strengthening, affording infant mobility [3,4]. Additionally, the infant's head position during sleep should be alternated on a nightly basis from left to right sides. The goal is to prevent the establishment of a persistent sleep position or "position of comfort" that, once established, can be exceedingly difficult to reverse. Infants should spend minimal time in car seats or other seating mechanisms that maintain supine positioning. By continuing to support "Back to Sleep" and incorporating these preventative measures, primary care providers can promote a new campaign: "Back to Sleep and Round Again" (M. Cunningham, Seattle Children's Hospital, Craniofacial Center, personal communication, 2003).

The true incidence of deformational plagiocephaly at an early age is probably underestimated. As the infant attains motor skills affording greater mobility, the deformation remodels, never coming to clinical attention or requiring intervention. As public awareness of deformational plagiocephaly increases, however, parents seek professional advice for this condition at an earlier age, allowing for the institution of behavioral modifications that have a significant likelihood of success. It has been the authors' experience that the two factors affecting the treatment plan and ultimate outcome for these patients are (1) the age at presentation and (2) the severity of the deformity. As the age at presentation increases and the severity of the deformity worsens, the potential for successful correction with behavioral modification alone decreases significantly. Although no universal treatment plan has been adopted, there is a general consensus on the approach to the child with deformational plagiocephaly. One such protocol, the "Decision Tree" designed by Cranial Technologies (Tempe, AZ) in 2002, has been published and is gaining favor (Fig. 9).

In the case of infants presenting with deformational plagiocephaly at less than 5 to 6 months of age, behavioral modifications or mechanical adjustments are initially implemented and given a chance to work.

These modifications focus on attempts at repositioning the infant's head during sleep. This repositioning can be performed with the placement of a rolled-up receiving blanket so that the rounded side of the head is dependent against the mattress, off-loading the affected side of the occiput. Parents are advised to alter the infant's position in the crib to encourage the spending of less time on the affected side. Because sleeping space is frequently against a room wall, the crib should be positioned so that the infant is forced to lie on the unaffected side to receive auditory and visual stimuli from toys, mobiles, and activity in the room. During feeding, parents are encouraged to position the infant so that the cradling arm removes pressure from the affected side of the skull rather than contributing to it. When the infant is awake, observed prone placement in the form of "tummy time" is recommended.

On initial evaluation of the infant, the physician takes care to note any evidence of head tilt or twist that would indicate muscular torticollis. If torticollis is diagnosed, neck exercises are performed in the office and should be taught to the parents as part of the management. If notable resistance is met on the first attempt to range the infant's neck, then a cervical spine series should be obtained to rule out a skeletal anomaly consistent with bony torticollis.

Neck exercises with each diaper change have been recommended [3]. These exercises entail gently rotating the child's head so that the chin touches the shoulder and holding for 10 seconds. This exercise is performed for three repetitions bilaterally, stretching the SCM muscle. The head is then tilted so that the ear touches the ipsilateral shoulder and again held for 10 seconds; this exercise is performed bilaterally for three repetitions, stretching the SCM and trapezius muscle. Chin-to-chest stretches complete the program. This exercise routine is estimated to take approximately 2 additional minutes per diaper change [3]. If the parents are simply unable to comply with these recommendations, a physical therapy (PT) consultation is obtained. The child is seen for follow-up after 1 month. If significant progress with the prescribed at-home PT treatments is not observed at this follow-up, then cervical spine films are obtained to rule out the skeletal anomalies of skeletal torticollis, and an ophthalmology consultation is obtained to rule out ocular torticollis. The vast majority of children with muscular torticollis associated with deformational plagiocephaly are successfully treated with home PT by the parents. It is exceedingly rare to find a patient with recalcitrant torticollis from a nonfunctional fibrotic SCM muscle requiring surgical release. Infants are monitored on a monthly basis

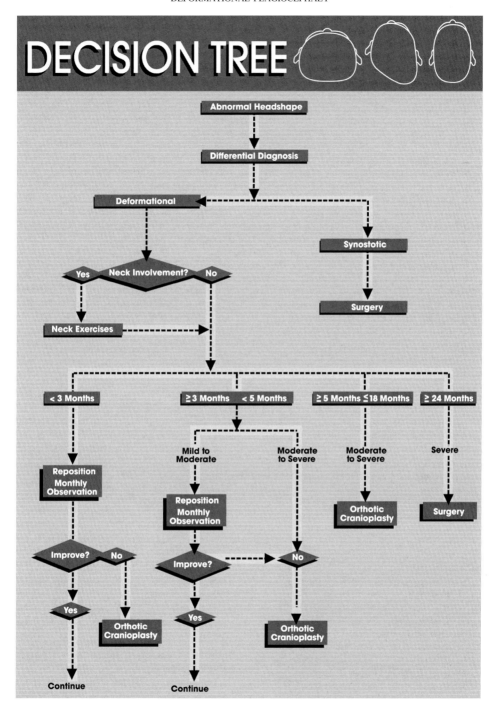

Fig. 9. Decision tree form for deformational plagiocephaly. (Courtesy of Cranial Technologies, 2002; with permission.)

until 5 to 6 months of age for evidence of success with behavioral modification and improvement of occipital deformity.

Those infants who at 5 to 6 months of life (1) fail conservative management, (2) present with initial moderate to severe deformities, or (3) have concomitant anterior craniofacial deformities are candidates for external cranioplasty with an orthotic device. These custom-fitted molding helmets facilitate skull reshaping (Fig. 10). The soft helmet is constructed after either obtaining a custom plaster mold of the infant's head or generating a CT scan. The typical cranial molding helmet is constructed with an outer shell of lightweight plastic and an inner layer of foam. It is fashioned in such a way that the device is snug where the head is prominent and hollow where the head is flat, allowing the rapidly growing brain to "push out" the deformed cranium and assume its normal morphology.

Typically, children with deformational plagiocephaly present to the craniofacial surgeon at approximately 6 months of life, having failed conservative therapy and developed an established sleep position [10,31]. Helmet therapy is started as soon as it becomes evident that conservative methods have failed or will not be an option because of severity or advanced age. Time is of the essence, because the goal is to capitalize on the still-malleable cranial bones. Many physicians observe optimal results when therapy is initiated between 6 and 8 months of age. When cranial molding-helmet therapy is started after the age of 12 months, remolding is less successful in the experience of most clinicians [10,31]. A compliant, dedicated caretaker is required for success

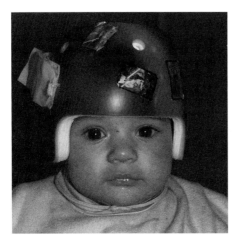

Fig. 10. Child with cranial molding helmet.

with this treatment, because older infants may not eagerly embrace the helmet at first. Initially, children go through a short "warm-up" period, then are quickly encouraged to spend at least 23 hours a day in the helmet. Consistency of helmet use directly correlates with final outcomes. When use is consistent, infants adapt with typical alacrity; they have even been reported to experience some separation angst when therapy is discontinued. Children are serially seen at 2- to 3-month intervals by the surgeon and receive a developmental and neurologic examination as well as an assessment of the remodeling progress. The child is seen every 1 to 2 weeks by the prosthetist, who adjusts the helmet, adding and removing inner foam padding where indicated, accommodating head growth and correction of the deformity.

Clarren et al [32] first proposed remolding the deformed skull with a helmet in 1979, and Levy concluded that nonoperative helmet therapy had an efficacy equivalent to operative treatment [4,31]. On August 31, 1998, the US Food and Drug Administration classified cranial orthotic devices as neurologic devices and approved them for use in infants 3 to 18 months of age with moderate to severe nonsynostotic deformational plagiocephaly. Many authors report improvements in cranial vault asymmetry in up to 40% to 60% of cases. Vies et al [33] prospectively evaluated 105 infants with deformational plagiocephaly and compared helmet therapy with repositioning therapy. Although improvement in cosmetic outcome was witnessed in both groups, contour improvement was far more impressive in the helmeted group. This prospective trial is consistent with other literature suggesting that orthotic helmet therapy results in a faster and better result than positional therapy alone, particularly in infants with severe deformities [10,31]. Average lengths of helmet therapy range from 4 to 5 months [10,31,33]. No study to date has identified significant complications of helmet therapy. The drawbacks described to parents usually include malodorous perspiration, minor skin irritations, nonreimbursable cost, and the stigma of helmet use. The surgical correction of true deformational plagiocephaly is rare and is usually reserved for those infants presenting with severe deformities and at an age when helmet therapy is not effective.

It has been the experience of the authors that third-party payers increasingly meet demands for reimbursement for treatment of deformational plagiocephaly with cranial molding helmets with resistance. Occasionally, reimbursement has been obtained for the infant with severe anterior craniofacial changes or functional components such as torticollis. Unfortunately, helmet therapy is a time-intensive endeavor for the prosthetist and hence can be a costly one, with the price ranging from $2000 to $5000 for a complete course. Occasionally, a child outgrows the initial helmet during a long course of treatment and requires a second orthotic, potentially adding to the cost of care. Some researchers have reported that most children with deformational plagiocephaly will ultimately achieve satisfactory correction with conservative management [34]. However, it has been the present authors' experience that not all children "self-correct"; they have evaluated a cohort of children aged 2 to 5 years who presented with persistent craniofacial asymmetries and would have benefited from intervention. Certainly, the infant who at 6 months of life remains in a persistent sleep position and has developed craniofacial asymmetry is at significant risk for not "self-correcting" and for experiencing progressive asymmetry that may result in permanent craniofacial deformities.

Summary

The "Back to Sleep" campaign has dramatically decreased the incidence of sudden infant death syndrome; however, its sequelae of deformational plagiocephaly have today reached epidemic proportions. In the last decade, we have learned to distinguish deformational plagiocephaly clinically from craniosynostosis, thereby preventing its unnecessary surgical correction. Primary care providers must increasingly be aware of this condition and, in turn, educate new parents about its prevention. Should preventative measures fail and infants develop persistent sleep patterns that result in craniofacial deformities, deformational plagiocephaly can be treated successfully with behavior modification or cranial molding-helmet therapy.

References

[1] Nichter LS, Persing JA, Horowitz JH, Morgan RF, Nichter MA, Edgerton MT. External cranioplasty: historical perspectives. Plast Reconstr Surg 1986; 77(2):325–32.

[2] Hanson M, Mulliken JB. Frontal plagiocephaly: diagnosis and treatment. Clin Plast Surg 1994;21(4): 543–53.

[3] Persing J, James H, Swanson J, Kattwinkel J. Prevention and management of positional skull deformities in infants. Pediatrics 2003;112(1):199–202.

[4] Gruss JS, Ellenbogen RG, Whelan MF. Lambdoid

synostosis and posterior plagiocephaly. In: Lin KY, Ogle RC, Jane JA, editors. Craniofacial Surgery: Science and Surgical Technique. Philadelphia: WB Saunders; 2002. p. 233–51.

[5] Balan P, Kushnerenko E, Sahlin P, Huotilainen M, Naatanen R, Hukki J. Auditory ERPs reveal brain dysfunction in infants with plagiocephaly. J Craniofac Surg 2002;13(4):520–5.

[6] Shahinian HK, Jaekle R, Suh RH, Jarrahy R, Aguilar VC, Soojian M. Obstetrical factors governing the etiopathogenesis of lambdoid synostosis. Am J Perinatol 1998;15(5):281–6.

[7] Warren SM, Greenwald JA, Spector JA, Bouletreau P, Mehrara BJ, Longaker MT. New developments in cranial suture research. Plast Reconstr Surg 2001; 107(2):523–40.

[8] Vernacchio L, Corwin MJ, Lesko SM, Vezina RM, Hunt CE, Hoffman HJ, et al. Sleep position of low birth weight infants. Pediatrics 2003;111(3):633–40.

[9] Corwin MJ, Lesko SM, Heeren T, Vezina RM, Hunt CE, Mandell F, et al. Secular changes in sleep position during infancy: 1995–1998. Pediatrics 2003;111(1): 52–60.

[10] Losee JE, Englert CJ, Hua LB, Lawrence RA. Factors impacting non-synostotic occipital plagiocephaly: a retrospective review of 105 cases at a children's hospital. Presented at the 20th Anniversary Meeting of the Northeastern Society of Plastic Surgeons. Baltimore (MD), October 2003.

[11] Littlefield TR, Beals SP, Manwaring KH, Pomatto JK, Joganic EF, Golden KA, et al. Treatment of craniofacial asymmetry with dynamic orthotic cranioplasty. J Craniofac Surg 1998;9:11–7.

[12] Mulliken JB, Vander Woude DL, Hansen M, LaBrie RA, Scott RM. Analysis of posterior plagiocephaly: deformational versus synostotic. Plast Reconstr Surg 1999;103(2):371–80.

[13] Chadduck WM, Kast J, Donahue DJ. The enigma of lambdoid positional molding. Pediatr Neurosurg 1997; 26:304–11.

[14] Pople IK, Sanford RA, Muhlbauer MS. Clinical presentation and management of 100 infants with occipital plagiocephaly. Pediatr Neurosurg 1996;25:1–6.

[15] Willinger M, Hoffman HJ, Kuo-Tsung W, Hou JR, Kessler RC, Ward SL, et al. Factors associated with the transition to nonprone sleep positions of infants in the United States. JAMA 1998;280(4): 329–46.

[16] Teighgraeber JF, Ault JK, Baumgartner J, Waller A, Messersmith M, Gateno J, et al. Deformational posterior plagiocephaly: diagnosis and treatment. Cleft Palate Craniofac J 2002;39(6):582–6.

[17] Kane AA, Mitchell LE, Craven KP, Marsh JL. Observations on a recent increase in plagiocephaly without synostosis. Pediatrics 1996;97:877–85.

[18] O'Broin ES, Allcutt C, Earley MJ. Posterior plagiocephaly: proactive conservative management. Br J Plast Surg 1999;52:18–23.

[19] Ellenbogen RG, Gruss JS, Cunningham M, Update on

craniofacial surgery: the differential diagnosis of lambdoid synostosis/posterior plagiocephaly. Clin Neurosurg 2000;43:303–18.

[20] Dias MS, Klein DM, Backstrom JW. Occipital plagiocephaly: deformation or lambdoid synostosis? Pediatr Neurosurg 1996;24:61–8.

[21] Roddi R, Jansen MA, Vaandrager JM, van der Meulen CH. Plagiocephaly—new classification and clinical study of a series of 100 patients. J Craniomaxillofac Surg 1995;23:347–54.

[22] Menard RM, David DJ. Unilateral lambdoid synostosis: morphological characteristics. J Craniofac Surg 1998;9(3):240–6.

[23] Losee JE, Bartlett SP, Feldman E, Ketkar M, Kirschner RE, Singh D, et al. Non-synostotic occipital plagiocephaly: radiographic diagnosis of the sticky suture. Presented at the 60th Anniversary Meeting of the American Cleft Palate-Craniofacial Association. Asheville (NC), April 2003.

[24] Cherney J, Beals S, Cohen S, Holmes R, Joganic E, Kelly K, et al. Evaluation of a new severity assessment scale for deformational plagiocephaly. Presented at the 61st Annual Meeting of the American Cleft Palate–Craniofacial Association. Chicago, March 15–20, 2004

[25] Francel P, Panchal J. Detection of visual field abnormalities in posterior plagiocephaly. Presented at the 61st Annual Meeting of the American Cleft Palate–Craniofacial Association. Chicago, March 15–20, 2004.

[26] Gupta PC, Foster J, Crowe S, Papay FA, Luciano M, Traboulsi ET. Ophthalmologic findings in patients with nonsyndromic plagiocephaly. J Craniofac Surg 2003; 14(4):529–32.

[27] Magge SH, Westerveld M, Pruzinsky T, Persing JA. Long-term neuropsychological effects of sagittal craniosynostosis on child development. J Craniofac Surg 2002;13(1):99–103.

[28] Virtanen R, Korhonen T, Fagerholm J, Viljanto J. Neurocognitive sequelae of scaphocephaly. Pediatrics 1999;103(4):791–5.

[29] Panchal J, Amirsheybani H, Gurwitch R, Cook V, Francel P, Neas B, et al. Neurodevelopment in children with single-suture craniosynostosis and plagiocephaly with synostosis. Plast Reconstr Surg 2001;108(6): 1492–500.

[30] Miller RI, Clarren SK. Long-term developmental outcomes in patients with deformational plagiocephaly. Pediatrics 2000;105(2):e26.

[31] Teighgraeber JF, Seymour-Dempse K, Baumgartner JE, Xia JJ, Waller A, Gateno J, et al. Molding helmet therapy in the treatment of brachycephaly and plagiocephaly. J Craniofac Surg 2004;15(1):118–23.

[32] Clarren SK, Smight DW, Hanson JW. Helmet treatment for plagiocephaly and congenital muscular torticollis. J Pediatr 1979;94:43–6.

[33] Vies JS, Colla C, Weber JW, Beuls E, Wilmin J, Kingma H. Helmet versus nonhelmet treatment in non synostotic positional posterior plagiocephaly. J Craniofac Surg 2000;11(6):572–4.

[34] David DJ, Menard RM. Occipital plagiocephaly. Br J Plast Surg 2000;53:367–77.

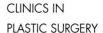

CLINICS IN
PLASTIC SURGERY

Clin Plastic Surg 32 (2005) 65 – 78

Treatment of pediatric breast problems

John A. van Aalst, MD[a],*, A. Michael Sadove, MD[b]

[a]*Division of Plastic and Reconstructive Surgery, University of North Carolina at Chapel Hill, CD# 7195, Suite 2100,
Bioinformatics Building, Chapel Hill, NC 27599, USA*
[b]*Division of Plastic Surgery, Riley Hospital for Children, Indiana University, Indianapolis, IN 46202-5124, USA*

Pediatric breast anomalies span a wide range of problems, some common, such as polythelia, that present as isolated abnormalities and others rare, such as amastia, that may present with a constellation of other abnormalities. Treatment of breast abnormalities involves decisions about type and timing of treatment, with a view to immediate and future aesthetic considerations. The authors have previously categorized breast anomalies as hyperplastic, deformational, and hypoplastic to facilitate discussion of pediatric breast anomalies [1]. Hyperplastic anomalies are characterized by excess breast tissue and include polythelia, polymastia, gynecomastia, juvenile hypertrophy, and giant fibroadenomas (Table 1). Treatment for these anomalies requires breast reduction techniques. Deformational anomalies, including iatrogenic and traumatic injuries to the breast, tend to have a paucity of breast tissue. These abnormalities may be secondary to tube thoracostomy, thoracotomy, and tumor removal or may follow burns and penetrating trauma. Deformational anomalies require a combination of staged releases to accommodate breast growth and augmentation procedures [1]. Hypoplastic anomalies, characterized by breast-tissue paucity, include hypoplasia, tuberous breast, Poland Syndrome, athelia, and amastia. These anomalies require staged augmentation procedures.

Breast development

The breast develops during the sixth week of gestation from an anlage of ectodermal cells along the "milk lines," or primitive mammary ridges. These ridges extend from the axilla to the groin. By the 10th week of gestation, the upper and lower parts of these ridges atrophy; the middle or pectoral ridges, at the level of the fourth interspace, persist and later develop into breast tissue. The areola develops in the fifth month of gestation, and the nipple appears shortly after birth [2].

Following birth, circulating maternal estrogens may result in breast-tissue enlargement. As maternal estrogens are metabolized, breast tissue involutes, remaining quiescent through childhood. At this time, the breast consists of epithelial-lined ducts with surrounding connective tissue. At the onset of puberty, hormonal influence results in breast-tissue growth: estrogens cause ductal and stromal tissue growth, and progesterone causes alveolar budding and lobular growth [3]. Breast growth begins with thelarche (which precedes puberty by approximately a year) at an average age of 11 but may have a normal range of 8 to 15. Breast development as described by Tanner [4] proceeds through stages I through V, with breast maturity represented by Stage V. Nipple size differentiation occurs between Tanner stages IV and V [5]. Breast growth may be variable but is generally complete by 16 to 18 years of age.

Aesthetic considerations

Because breast growth may be variable and asymmetric, even in normal individuals, it is incum-

* Corresponding author.
E-mail address: john_vanaalst@med.unc.edu
(J.A. van Aalst).

0094-1298/05/$ – see front matter © 2005 Elsevier Inc. All rights reserved.
doi:10.1016/j.cps.2004.08.005

Table 1
Categories of pediatric breast anomalies [1]

| | Deformational | | |
| | --- | | |
Hyperplastic	Iatrogenic	Traumatic	Hypoplastic
Polythelia	Thoracostomy	Burns	Hypoplasia
Polymastia	Thoracotomy	Penetrating	Tuberous breast
Symmastia	Tumor excision		Poland syndrome
Gynecomastia			Athelia
Giant fibroadenoma			Amazia
Pediatric hyperplasia			Amastia
Juvenile hypertrophy			

bent on the surgeon to delay surgery of the breast until breast development is complete [6]. An estimate of completion of breast growth may be elicited from the patient or patient's family by asking whether the patient's bra size has changed in the previous year. If it has not changed, breast development is probably complete. Because many breast anomalies result in asymmetric growth of the breasts, allowing the normal (or more normal) breast to reach maturity gives the surgeon a template for achieving breast symmetry. Operating on a growing breast may result in unnecessary revisional surgery following complete growth of the breast.

Hyperplastic breast abnormalities

Hyperplastic breast anomalies are characterized by excessive breast tissue. One of the most common congenital anomalies of the breast is polythelia, the presence of supernumerary nipples or nipple-areolar complexes. The condition may occur in both males and females [7,8] and has a reported incidence as high as 5.6% [7]. The condition usually occurs sporadically and in rare instances may be associated

with nephro-urologic anomalies [9]; familial cases have also been reported. Polythelia may occur at any point along the embryonic milk line from the axilla to the groin (Fig. 1A). Pigmented lesions within these embryonic lines should be excised before puberty; after the onset of puberty in females, resection may require wider tissue excision because of glandular growth. Cancerous degeneration of the accessory nipple-areolar complex has been reported and provides additional justification for excision of these lesions [7]. Elliptic excision of the nipple-areolar complex is usually sufficient for removal. If multiple nipple-areolar complexes occur on the breast itself (Fig. 1B), it may be challenging to determine which nipple-areolar complex is associated with glandular/ductal tissue. An MRI may be needed to determine which nipple-areolar complex to preserve.

Polymastia, a more rare condition than polythelia, may also occur anywhere along the embryonic milk line [8]. This condition usually occurs sporadically, but familial cases have been reported; latent cases may become noticeable during puberty, pregnancy, or lactation. Polymastia can occur as an isolated finding or present with congenital renal anomalies [10]. Treatment requires removal of the accessory gland,

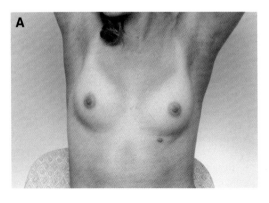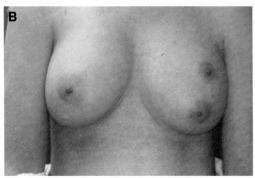

Fig. 1. (*A*) An accessory nipple located in the inframammary fold of the left breast. (*B*) An accessory nipple-areolar complex on the left breast.

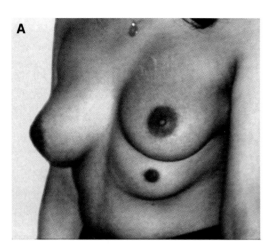
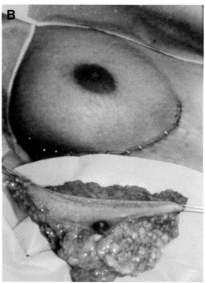

Fig. 2. (*A*) An accessory left breast in an adolescent patient. (*B*) Excision of the accessory gland and primary closure were performed.

with primary closure (Fig. 2). Further follow-up is required because of the possibility of developing cancer in any retained breast tissue.

Symmastia, a condition of medial confluence of the breasts, may be either congenital or iatrogenic (following breast reduction). The entity was first described by Spence et al [11] in 1983. He proposed two methods of correcting the medial web: using an inferiorly based triangular skin flap advanced superiorly in a V-Y fashion or, in an attempt to place the scar below the sternum, using a superiorly-based medial flap to fill in the defect after web excision. More recently, authors have suggested a periareolar approach to the symmastic breast, with use of dermal plication sutures to redrape the presternal breast web over the sternal periosteum. Suction-assisted lipectomy can be used to debulk excess fat in the breast web [12].

Another common form of hyperplasia confronting the pediatric plastic surgeon is gynecomastia, which affects up to 65% of males aged 14 to 15 years. Gynecomastia is initially characterized by proliferation of fibroblastic stroma and ducts and generally resolves spontaneously without the need for surgical intervention [13]. If the condition persists beyond a year, fibrosis and hyalinization occur with regression of epithelial proliferation, increasing the likelihood that surgical intervention will be required. Surgical therapy for gynecomastia depends on the extent of breast tissue and the degree of ptosis [14]. Simon et al [14] proposed a three-grade classification system for gynecomastia, in which Grade 1 is characterized by slight breast enlargement without skin redundancy (Table 2). Grade 2a is characterized by moderate breast enlargement without skin redundancy, Grade 2b by moderate breast enlargement with marked skin redundancy, and Grade 3 by both marked breast enlargement and skin redundancy. Timing for surgical intervention is based on the absence of an endocrine causative agent for the gynecomastia, the persistence of the breast enlargement for longer than a year, and the social stigma encountered by the patient.

The authors prefer to use a semicircular, periareolar incision for glandular resection and to use ultrasonic liposuction (US) in patients with grades 2a, 2b, and 3 gynecomastia. Before the advent of US,

Table 2
Gynecomastia grades and treatment preferences [14]

Grade I	Slight breast enlargement	No skin redundancy
Grade IIa	Moderate breast enlargement	No skin redundancy
Grade IIb	Moderate breast enlargement	Marked skin redundancy
Grade III	Marked breast enlargement	Marked skin redundancy

skin incisions used to excise excess skin resulted in unacceptable chest-wall scars. US has made possible increased breast-volume reduction without an added scar burden. The US trochar is introduced through a small stab incision in the proximal anterior axillary line and provides access to tissue not directly excised through the periareolar incision. Contour irregularities secondary to edema and seroma usually resolve without the need for additional intervention (Fig. 3). In cases of persistent skin excess, a circumareolar incision may be required to resect skin; however, this is only done as a secondary, staged procedure.

Giant fibroadenomas are benign, discrete lesions that present during puberty as unilateral, rapidly growing breast masses (Fig. 4). The lesion is the result of breast-tissue hypersensitivity to normal levels of gonadal hormones. Diagnosis is made by breast-tissue biopsy. Treatment involves conservative breast-reduction techniques [15]. Timing for surgery is dictated by the onset of the rapid growth phase of

the fibroadenoma; surgery may need to precede complete breast development because of the development of gross asymmetry in breast size.

Pediatric hyperplasia of the breast or juvenile hypertrophy is rare and has an unknown etiology. It is not associated with any endocrine abnormalities, and the patient otherwise exhibits normal growth. The goal of surgery is volume reduction with symmetric breast size and anatomically correct nipple-areolar location (Fig. 5). Prepubertal hypertrophy (which is usually bilateral) and virginal hypertrophy (which develops after puberty and may be either unilateral or bilateral) are also treated with breast-reduction techniques. Classes of asymmetry in hyperplasia include unilateral hyperplasia, bilateral symmetric hyperplasia, and a combination of hypertrophy and hypoplasia [16]. Treatment involves a combination of reduction techniques (the authors prefer an inferior pedicle technique), which may require resection of differential amounts of tissue to achieve breast

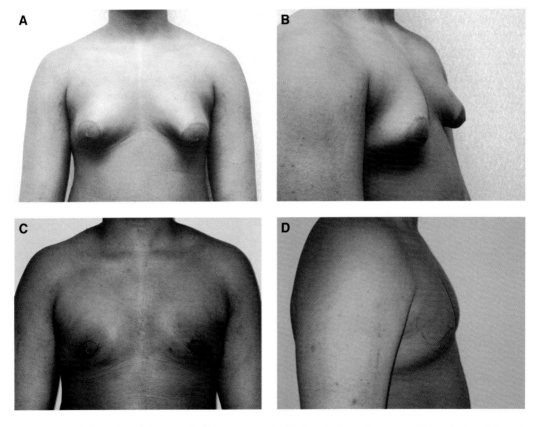

Fig. 3. (A) Frontal view of an adolescent male with gynecomastia. (B) Lateral view of the same patient. (C) Frontal view after glandular excision using a semicircular, periareolar incision with ultrasonic liposuction. No skin was excised. (D) Postoperative lateral view of same patient.

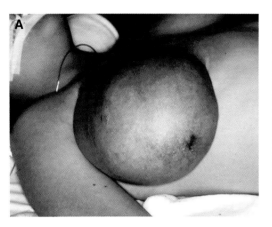
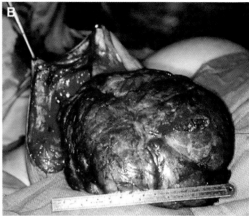

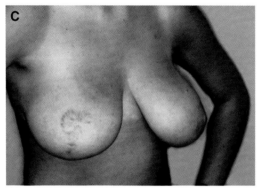

Fig. 4. (*A*) Intraoperative view of a giant fibroadenoma of the right breast. (*B*) Fibroadenoma specimen before final excision. (*C*) The same patient following excision of the fibroadenoma.

symmetry. Surgery should be delayed until the end of puberty when breast growth is complete; otherwise, unnecessary revisions may be required because of continued breast growth.

Deformational breast anomalies

Injury to the breast nearly always results in a hypoplastic deformity, with a combination of deficiencies in skin, nipple-areola, or glandular tissue. Scar burden at the injury site tethers the breast tissue to the chest wall, resulting in a contour deformity.

Iatrogenic anomalies

One of the more common pediatric breast injuries is secondary to tube thoracostomy placement. The thoracostomy site develops a scar and fibrous tract that tethers breast tissue to the chest wall, leading to a localized contour deformity. These patients require release of the fibrous tract to accommodate normal breast growth during puberty. No further intervention is usually required.

Females who have undergone previous thoracotomy may similarly have breast tissue tethered to the anterior chest wall; violation of the breast bud by the initial thoracotomy incision may also result in breast hypoplasia (Fig. 6). Treatment of patients with previous anterolateral thoracotomy necessitates release of the scar tissue tethering the breast to the chest wall. Breast hypoplasia, which may be either segmental or total, requires breast-mound reconstruction with implant placement. Heightened awareness of breast hypoplasia after anterolateral thoracotomy has led some authors to suggest that a posterior thoracotomy be used instead of an anterolateral thoracotomy [17].

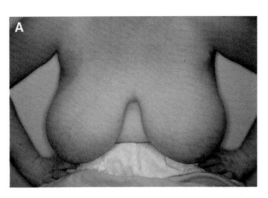
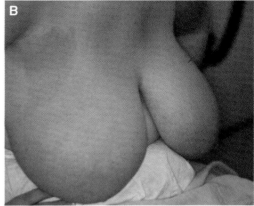
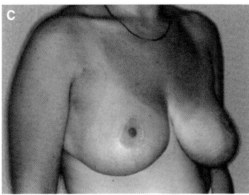

Fig. 5. (*A*) A patient with pediatric juvenile hypertrophy. (*B*) Oblique view of same patient. (*C*) Postoperative oblique view following reduction mammoplasty.

Tumor excision

Tumors of the pediatric breast are generally benign [18–20], although they may rarely be malignant [21–23]. In a series assessing 64 pediatric and adolescent patients with palpable breast lesions, the causes included gynecomastia, cysts, fibroadenomas, lymph nodes, galactoceles, duct ectasia, and infection. No malignancies were noted [24]. In another series of 27 pediatric breast tumors that required excision, 26 were benign and one was a metastatic carcinoma to the breast [25]. Although the pediatric plastic surgeon is unlikely to be the primary surgeon excising these breast lesions, he or she is the one who will be called on to treat the sequelae of their resection. If these tumors were excised before breast development, a possibility exists that the breast bud may have been injured; even without direct injury to the breast bud, scar tissue surrounding the breast may constrict breast development. A patient with a childhood hemangioma of the left breast underwent resection of the lesion and subsequently developed a contour irregularity of the left breast that was treated by scar-tissue release combined with breast augmentation (Fig. 7).

Traumatic anomalies

The burned breast is a particularly difficult challenge to the pediatric plastic surgeon. During acute excision and grafting, the breast bud must be protected. If the breast requires skin grafting, sheet grafts should be considered to improve cosmesis. During puberty, as the breast grows, conservative treatment is advised. If the breast bud is not injured during management of the initial burn, breast growth will occur but may be hindered by scar contractures (Fig. 8). Z-plasties and scar contracture release with additional skin grafting with unmeshed sheets may be

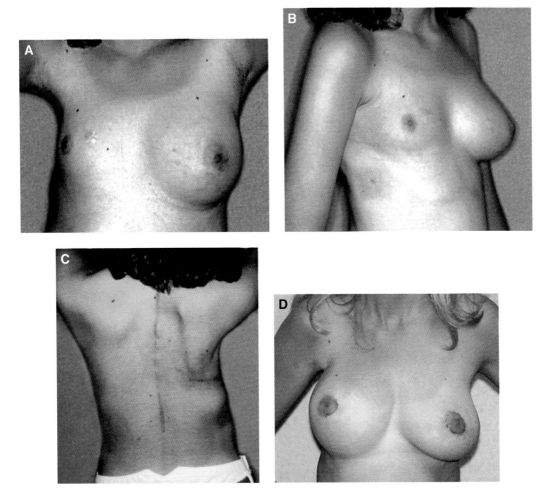

Fig. 6. (*A*) A frontal view of right breast hypoplasia after anterolateral thoracotomy. (*B*) Oblique view of same patient. (*C*) Posterior view of the thoracotomy scar. (*D*) The same patient after augmentation mammoplasty.

required to accommodate breast growth. Breast hypoplasia will result if the breast bud is injured during the initial burn. These patients require breast mound reconstruction with tissue expanders, followed by placement of a submuscular implant (Fig. 9). If the contralateral breast has not been injured, it may be used as a template for reconstruction of the injured breast. Nipple-areolar–complex reconstruction with skin-graft or tattooing techniques may be performed after breast reconstruction has been completed [26]. Long-term follow-up of the patient is required.

Penetrating trauma to the breast presents a problem similar to the iatrogenic breast problems caused by tube thoracostomy or thoracotomy. Cor-

rection requires release of the fibrous connections between the breast and chest wall, followed by breast reconstruction using implants as needed. The time for surgical intervention is usually during puberty, when breast asymmetry becomes accentuated with growth of the normal breast. Revisions may be required if breast growth is not complete at the time of the initial intervention.

Hypoplastic breast abnormalities

Breast hypoplasia (with an intact nipple-areolar complex) may be either unilateral or bilateral. Treat-

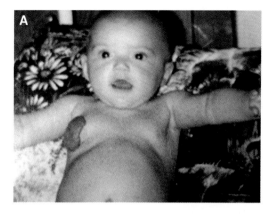
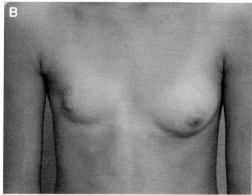
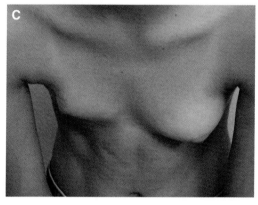

Fig. 7. (*A*) Right breast hemangioma in an infant. (*B,C*) Contour deformity of the right breast becoming more noticeable during adolescence.

ment requires single-breast augmentation mammoplasty in unilateral hypoplasia (Fig. 10), whereas bilateral asymmetric hypoplasia may require differential augmentation of the two breasts [27].

The tuberous breast deformity is characterized by breast hypoplasia, including a deficiency in base diameter, breast tissue herniation into the areola, deficient skin envelope, and elevation of the inframammary fold [28]. Several classification systems have been developed to describe the tuberous breast [28–30]. The three-tier system proposed by Meara et al [30] is the most utilitarian. The Type I tuberous breast has medial quadrant hypoplasia, Type II has lower medial and lateral quadrant hypoplasia, and Type III has severe breast constriction (Table 3). Increasing grade of tuberous breast deformity involves a progressive elevation of the inframammary fold, an increasing paucity of skin, a decreasing breast volume, and increasing ptosis. Unfavorable characteristics for reconstruction with an implant include a short inframammary fold–to–nipple distance and a constricted breast base that does not

easily accommodate an implant. To treat the abnormality, the breast base needs to be expanded, the inframammary fold needs to be lowered, breast volume needs to be increased, and ptosis must be corrected. In more severe deformities, division of breast tissue is required to increase the breast base, but an attractive outcome is difficult to obtain. More favorable characteristics in tuberous breast include a broader breast base that adequately covers an implant and a greater inframammary fold–to–nipple distance, allowing simple release of breast-tissue herniation into the nipple-aerolar complex. Outcomes in these cases are more favorable (Fig. 11).

Although the correction of tuberous breast deformity has leaned heavily on the use of implant augmentation, some authors prefer to use inferiorly based flaps for reconstruction of breast contour [31]. This technique results in a smaller breast and is appropriate for less severe cases of tuberous breast deformity. Tissue-expansion techniques may also be used to expand the base circumference of the breast. At an initial procedure, the expander is placed in

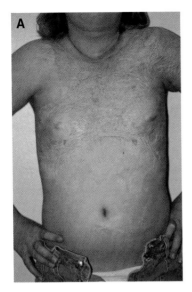
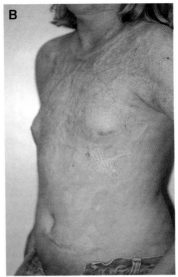
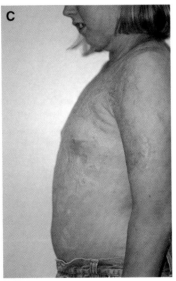

Fig. 8. Bilateral breast burns. (*A*) Anterior view of a prepubescent female. (*B*) Oblique view of the same patient with breast bud growth, and (*C*) lateral view. (Courtesy of C.S. Hultman, MD, University of North Carolina, Chapel Hill.)

either a subglandular or submuscular position through an inframammary incision. During expansion, the base circumference of the breast and the skin envelope are expanded; the position of the inframammary fold is simultaneously lowered. At a second procedure, the expander is exchanged for a permanent implant, tissue herniation into the areola is corrected, the areola itself is reduced, and a mastopexy is performed [32].

Another form of breast hypoplasia is Poland syndrome. Poland's initial description of the defor-

mity that bears his name included absence of the pectoralis major and minor muscles and syndactyly of the ipsilateral hand [33]. The full spectrum of the anomaly—in addition to those characteristics initially noted by Poland—includes absence of multiple ribs with chest-wall depression, athelia or amastia, absence of axillary hair, limited subcutaneous chest-wall fat, and brachy-syndactyly. The anomaly occurs in 1 in 20,000 to 30,000 live births; it may be unilateral [34] or more rarely bilateral [34,35], sporadic or familial [36]. Treatment options for the

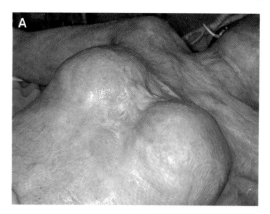
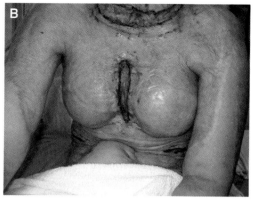

Fig. 9. (*A*) Bilateral submuscular implants in a patient with breast burns. (*B*) Scar contracture release with placement of split-thickness skin graft. (Courtesy of J. J. Coleman III, MD, R. Sood, MD, Indiana University Medical Center, Indianapolis, IN.)

breast and chest-wall anomalies include autologous tissue [37], pedicled (latissimus or rectus abdominis) or free (rectus abdominis) musculocutaneous flaps, and synthetic materials [38], alone or in combination. The authors prefer to correct the defect with a latissimus dorsi flap and placement of a breast implant (Fig. 12). Some authors have advocated the use of endoscopy to assist in the harvest and placement of the latissimus dorsi flap [39], but the present authors have found that a small incision suffices for harvest and placement of the flap, obviating endoscopic instrumentation. Once harvested, the latissimus flap must be fastidiously inset along the infraclavicular margin to prevent dehisence, which may result in recurrent contour deformities. The authors' preference for the latissimus dorsi flap was born out of the observation of high reopera-

tion rates among patients undergoing synthetic chest-wall reconstruction without myocutaneous flap coverage [1].

An entity separate from Poland's anomaly, referred to as anterior thoracic hypoplasia, has recently been reported [40]. These patients have a unilateral sunken chest wall, hypoplasia of the breast, and a superiorly displaced nipple-areola complex; significantly, they have a normal sternal position and a normal pectoralis muscle. Augmentation mammoplasty alone has been used successfully to treat these individuals.

Athelia (absence of the nipple) (Fig. 13), amazia (absence of the mammary gland), and amastia (absence of nipple and gland) are rare congenital hypoplastic anomalies [41,42]. Breast absence is defined by absence of the nipple. According to Lin

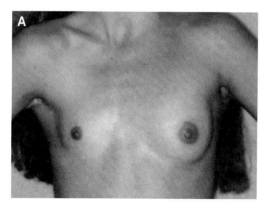
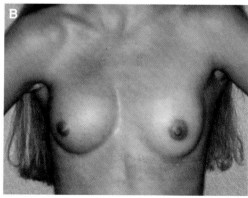

Fig. 10. (*A*) A patient with unilateral hypoplasia of the right breast. (*B*) The same patient after left breast augmentation with an implant.

Table 3
Grades of tuberous breast [30]

	Type I	Type II	Type III
Base	Minor constriction	Moderate constriction	Severe constriction
Inframammary fold	Normal	Medial elevation; minor lateral elevation	Substantial elevation of entire fold
Skin envelope	Sufficient	Inferior insufficiency	Circumferential insufficiency
Volume	Adequate	Mild/moderate deficiency	Severe deficiency
Ptosis	None	Minimal/moderate	Severe

et al [42], there are three groups of patients with amastia: those with bilateral absence of the breast secondary to congenital ectodermal defects, those with unilateral absence of the breast (a variant of Poland syndrome), and those with bilateral absence of the breast. Amastia that is associated with congenital ectodermal defects affects both males and females; it is associated with abnormalities of the skin and its appendages, the teeth and nails. Bilateral absence of the breast may occur as an isolated abnormality or may be associated with palate and upper-extremity anomalies. The defect may be sporadic or familial [42].

Construction of the breast mound in patients with amastia may be accomplished with tissue expansion and subsequent implant placement [42] but should be undertaken with caution because of possible aberrancies in the blood supply to the skin [43]. The breast mound may also be created with autologous tissue, including transverse rectus abdominis or latissimus dorsi myocutaneous flaps. Free-flap reconstruction with transverse rectus abdominis has also been described [44]. Tissue transfer avoids the problem of anomalous blood supply to the chest-wall skin. However, both implant and autologous mammoplasty face the challenge of appropriate creation of the

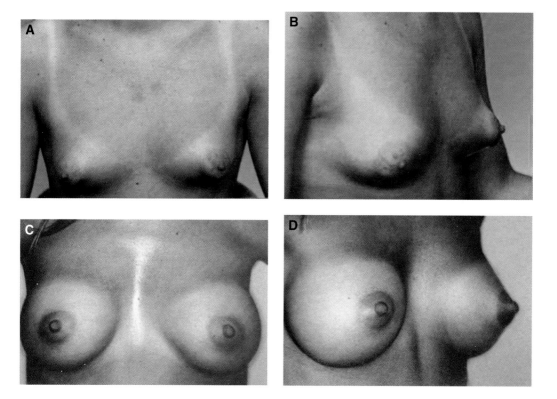

Fig. 11. (*A*) A patient with bilateral tuberous breast deformity. (*B*) Oblique view of same patient. (*C*) Frontal view following release of breast-tissue herniation into the nipple-areolar complex and bilateral augmentation mammoplasty. (*D*) Oblique view after augmentation mammoplasty.

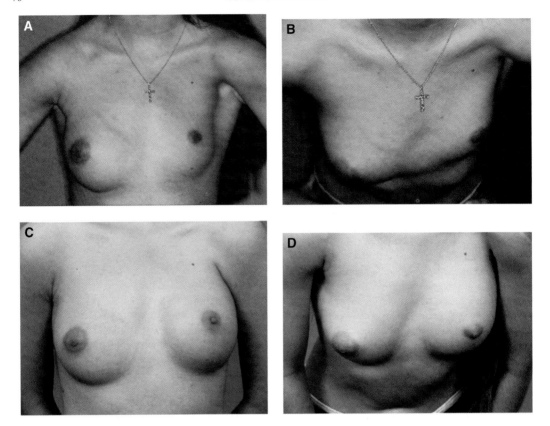

Fig. 12. (*A*) Poland's syndrome with left breast hypoplasia. (*B*) Absence of the pectoralis major in same patient. (*C*) Postoperative frontal view of patient after reconstruction with latissimus dorsi flap to the left breast. (*D*) Postoperative frontal view showing improved soft tissue contour under the left clavicle.

inframammary fold, owing to an absence of customary landmarks.

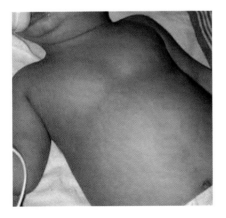

Fig. 13. A male infant with athelia.

Summary

Pediatric breast anomalies are common and wide-ranging in presentation. Categorizing these anomalies into the broad groups of hyperplastic, deformational, and hypoplastic anomalies facilitates discussion about treatment options and outcomes. Hyperplastic breast abnormalities benefit from a variety of reduction techniques. Deformational anomalies tend to require scar-tissue release and augmentation with both autologous and implant mammoplasty. Hypoplastic anomalies require augmentation mammoplasties. The classification of pediatric breast abnormalities, with due consideration given to surgical timing and the need for staged operations, aids in anticipating and optimizing clinical outcomes.

References

[1] Sadove AM, van Aalst JA. Congenital and acquired pediatric breast anomalies: a review of twenty years' experience. Plast Reconstr Surg, in press.

[2] Greydanus DE, Parks DS, Farrell EG. Breast disorders in children and adolescents. Ped Clin N Am 1989; 36(3):601–38.

[3] Pietsch J. Breast disorders. In: Lavery JP, Sanfilippo JS, editors. Pediatric and adolescent obstetrics and gynecology. New York: Springer-Verlag; 1985. p. 96–104.

[4] Tanner J. Growth at adolescence. Oxford (UK): Blackwell Scientific Publications; 1962.

[5] Rohn RD. Nipple (papilla) development in puberty: longitudinal observations in girls. Pediatrics 1987;79: 745–7.

[6] Stal S, Peterson R, Spira M. Aesthetic considerations and the pediatric population. Clin Plast Surg 1990; 17:133–49.

[7] Schmidt H. Supernumerary nipples: prevalence, size, sex and side predilection—a prospective clinical study. Eur J Pediatr 1998;157(10):821–3.

[8] Gilmore HT, Milroy M, Mello BJ. Supernumerary nipples and accessory breast tissue. S D J Med 1996; 49(5):149–51.

[9] Casey HD, Chasan PE, Chick LR. Familial polythelia without associated anomalies. Ann Plast Surg 1996; 36(1):101–4.

[10] Grossl NA. Supernumerary breast tissue: historical perspectives and clinical features. South Med J 2000; 93(1):29–32.

[11] Spence RJ, Feldman JJ, Ryan JJ. Symmastia: the problem of medial confluence of the breasts. Plast Reconstr Surg 1984;73(2):261–9.

[12] Salgado CJ, Mardini S. Periareolar approach for the correction of congenital symmastia. Plast Reconstr Surg 2004;113(3):992–4.

[13] Mathur R, Braunstein GD. Gynecomastia: pathomechanisms and treatment strategies. Horm Res 1997;48(3): 95–102.

[14] Simon BE, Kahn S. Classification and surgical correction of gynecomastia. Plast Reconstr Surg 1973;51: 48–52.

[15] Simmons RM, Cance WG, Iacicca MV. A giant juvenile fibroadenoma in a 12-year-old girl: a case for breast conservation. Breast J 2000;6(6):418–20.

[16] Malata CM, Boot JC, Bradbury ET, Ramli AR, Aharpe DT. Congenital breast asymmetry: subjective and objective assessment. Br J Plast Surg 1994;47(2): 95–102.

[17] Bleiziffer S, Schreiber C, Burgkart R, et al. The influence of right anterolateral thoracotomy in prepubescent female patients on late breast development and the incidence of scoliosis. J Thorac Cardiovasc Surg 2004; 127(5):1474–80.

[18] Sugai M, Murata K, Kimura N, Munakata H, Hada R, Kamata Y. Adenoma of the nipple in an adolescent. Breast Cancer 2002;9(3):254–6.

[19] Hsieh SC, Chen KC, Chu CC, Chou JM. Juvenile papillomatosis of the breast in a 9-year-old girl. Pediatr Surg Int 2001;17(2–3):206–8.

[20] Selamzde M, Gidener C, Koyuncuoglu M, Mevsim A. Borderline phylloides tumor in an 11-year-old girl. Pediatr Surg Int 1999;15:427–8.

[21] Binokay F, Soyupak SK, Inal M, et al. Primary and metastatic rhabdomyosarcoma in the breast: report of two pediatric cases. Eur J Radiol 2003;48(3):282–4.

[22] Murphy JJ, Morzaria S, Gow KW, Magee JF. Breast cancer in a 6-year-old child. J Pediatr Surg 2000;35(5): 765–7.

[23] Di Noto A, Paecheco BP, Vicala R, Itala J, Pellegrino J, Mendez RJ. Two cases of breast lymphoma mimicking juvenile hypertrophy. J Pediatr Adolesc Gynecol 1999; 12(1):33–5.

[24] Weinstein SP, Conant EF, Orel SG, Zuckerman JA, Bellah R. Spectrum of US findings in pediatric and adolescent patients with palpable breast masses. Radiographics 2000;20:1613–21.

[25] Ciftci AO, Tanyel FC, Buyukpamukcu N, Hicsonmez A. Female breast masses during childhood: a 25-year review. Eur J Pediatr Surg 1998;8(2):67–70.

[26] MacLennan SE, Wells MD, Neale HW. Reconstruction of the burned breast. Clin Plast Surg 2000;27(1): 123–9.

[27] Smith DJ, Palin WE, Katch V, Bennett JE. Surgical treatment of congenital breast asymmetry. Ann Plast Surg 1986;47:92–101.

[28] Rees TD, Aston S. The tuberous breast. Clin Plast Surg 1976;3:339–46.

[29] Von Heimburn D, Exner K, Kruft S, Lemperle S. The tuberous breast deformity: classification and treatment. Br J Plast Surg 1996;49(6):339–45.

[30] Meara JG, Kokker A, Bartlett G, Theile R, Mutimer K, Holmes AD. Tuberous breast deformity: principles and practice. Ann Plast Surg 2000;4S(L):607–11.

[31] Ribeiro L, Canzi W, Buss A, Accorsi Jr A. Tuberous breast: a new approach. Plast Reconstr Surg 1998;101: 42–50.

[32] Versaci AD, Rozzelle AA. Treatment of tuberous breasts utilizing tissue expansion. Aesthetic Plast Surg 1991;15(4):307–12.

[33] Poland A. Deficiency of the pectoral muscles. Guys Hosp Rep 1841;6:191.

[34] Shamberger RC, Welch KJ, Upton III J. Surgical treatment of thoracic deformity in Poland's syndrome. J Pediatr Surg 1989;24(8):760–5.

[35] Karnak I, Tanyel FC, Tuncbilek E, Unsal M, Buyukpamukcu N. Bilateral Poland anomaly. Am J Med Genet 1998;75(5):505–7.

[36] Shalev SA, Hall JG. Poland anomaly—report of an unusual family. Am J Med Genet 2003;118A(2):180–3.

[37] Longaker MT, Glat PM, Colen LB, Siebert JW. Reconstruction of breast asymmetry in Poland's chestwall deformity using microvascular free flaps. Plast Reconstr Surg 1997;99(2):429–36.

[38] Marks MW, Iacobucci J. Reconstruction of congenital chest wall deformities using solid silicone onlay prostheses. Chest Surg Clin N Am 2000;10(2):341–55.

[39] Borschel GH, Izenberg PH, Cederna PS. Endoscopi-
cally assisted reconstruction of male and female Poland
syndrome. Plast Reconstr Surg 2002;109:1536–43.

[40] Spear SL, Pelletiere CV, Lee ES, Grotting JC. Anterior
thoracic hypoplasia: a separate entity from Poland syndrome. Plast Reconstr Surg 2004;113(1):69–77.

[41] Trier WC. Complete breast absence. Plast Reconstr
Surg 1965;36:430–9.

[42] Lin KY, Nguyen DB, Williams RM. Complete breast
absence revisited. Plast Reconstr Surg 2000;106(1):
98–101.

[43] Taylor GA. Reconstruction of congenital amastia with
complication. Ann Plast Surg 1979;2(6):531–4.

[44] Tvrdek M, Kletensky J, Svoboda S. Aplasia of the
breast—reconstruction using a free tram flap. Acta
Chir Plast 2001;43(2):39–41.

ELSEVIER
SAUNDERS

CLINICS IN
PLASTIC SURGERY

Clin Plastic Surg 32 (2005) 79 – 98

Management of infant brachial plexus injuries

Saleh M. Shenaq, MD[a,b,*], Jamal M. Bullocks, MD[a,b],
Gupreet Dhillon, MD[a,b], Rita T. Lee, MD[a], John P. Laurent, MD[a,b]

[a]Texas Children's Hospital, 6701 Fannin Street Houston, TX 77030, USA
[b]Baylor College of Medicine, 6560 Fannin, #800, Houston, TX 77030, USA

Descriptions of injuries to the brachial plexus date back to references in *The Iliad* and the Old Testament [1–3]. Early documentations of upper extremity dysfunction, predominantly caused by obstetric manipulation and trauma, parallel those of the modern era. The first surgical descriptions of brachial plexus injury are attributed to Smellie in 1768 and Flaubert in 1827 [4,5]. Smellie discussed the significance of brachial plexus injury secondary to difficult obstetric manipulation. Flaubert is credited with one of the first anatomic descriptions of upper extremity paralysis secondary to cervical root avulsion and cord compression from industrial trauma.

In the late nineteenth century, Duchenne [6] contrived a schematic representation of the plexus injuries that conferred specific types of muscle paralysis of the arm. This work was further elaborated by Erb, Seeligmuller, and Klumpke [7–9] in 1874, with electrical stimulation studies that localized lesions to either the upper or the lower cervical roots. In 1900, Thorburn first performed surgical repair for traumatic rupture of cord elements [10]. This procedure was followed in 1920 by Wyeth and Taylor [11,12], who reported a large series of primary repairs of obstetric lesions.

Nevertheless, because the early cases of the twentieth century were characterized by an inability to measure outcomes, difficulties in diagnosis, and high perioperative morbidity, surgical repair subsequently fell out of favor. A renewed interest in the surgical treatment of brachial plexus injuries emerged during the First and Second World Wars, owing to the vast number of soldiers who endured brachial plexus injuries and the advances in surgical technique during that era. In 1947, H. J. Seddon [13] made the first attempts at surgical repair of injuries with nerve grafts; he published the first case of active flexion restoration with intercostal neurotization in 1963.

In 1957, Sydney Sunderland [1] published a comprehensive description of the complex anatomic considerations in brachial plexus injuries. The pioneering work of these two surgeons has defined the major strategies for managing peripheral nerve injury today. Over the last few decades, the contributions of Leffert, Narakas, Millesi, Terzis, Mackinnon, and others [14–21] have resulted in reproducible algorithms for the evaluation and treatment of both traumatic and obstetric brachial plexus injuries. The contemporary-setting large-scale studies by Gilbert, Boome, Shenaq, Laurent, Terzis, Wei, Clarke, and others [21–31] have demonstrated the benefit of microsurgical and secondary reconstruction in mitigating the functional deficits of obstetric brachial plexus palsy.

Epidemiology

Obstetric brachial plexus palsy (OBPP) occurs in 0.4 to 3 per 1000 term births [4,32–34]. In a large study of a million deliveries, Gilbert et al [35] determined that the risk factors for OBPP included gestational diabetes, forceps delivery, vacuum extrac-

* Corresponding author. Division of Plastic Surgery, Baylor College of Medicine, 6560 Fannin, #800, Houston, TX 77030.

E-mail address: sshenaq@bcm.tmc.edu (S.M. Shenaq).

0094-1298/05/$ – see front matter © 2005 Elsevier Inc. All rights reserved.
doi:10.1016/j.cps.2004.09.001

tion, and shoulder dystocia. Additionally, Jennett and other investigators [36–41] have found breech delivery, multiparity, macrosomia, and history of a previous child with brachial plexus injury to be independent risk factors for injury.

Erb-Duchenne palsy, the clinical presentation of upper cervical root injury, is seen in the majority of the cases [37,38,40–43]. In the authors' experience at Texas Children's Hospital, 73% of cases present as injuries to the upper cervical roots. The second most common cause is total plexus injuries, which account for 25% of cases. Isolated lower plexus injury or Klumpke palsy is rare (2%). Right-sided lesions are more common; bilateral injury occurs 4% of the time (a finding similar to that of widely published reports) and correlates with breech presentations [29,32,34, 39–46].

Mechanism of brachial plexus injury

Stretch, compression, and crush of brachial plexus components lead to neurologic deficits. Initially, the degree of neurologic deficit will depend on the anatomic location and the extent of the injury. In accordance with the properties of central nervous system plasticity, the long-term disability will depend on the type of nerve injury. Depending on the vector of the forces applied, injury can occur at the level of the roots, trunk, cords, or any combination of these.

Mechanical forces (traction, compression, and crush) can disrupt electrophysiologic and mechanical properties of the nerves, even in the presence of physical continuity of the nerve trunk. Extreme movements of the upper extremity result in an increase in scapulo-humeral angle that has the potential to lead to various grades of nerve injury, from simple neuropraxia to axonotmesis. The mobility of the cervical spine and the shoulder demands that the brachial plexus be flexible and able to undergo significant excursion without injury. The viscoelastic properties of peripheral nerves, the undulating course of fibers in the fascicles, and laxity on the perineurium and the mesoneurium provide the brachial plexus with flexibility and robustness, as required for a normal range of cervical spine and shoulder joint movements.

At the level of the vertebral foramina, anterior and posterior rootlets are covered by a sheath of dura. This dural sheath, together with transverse radicular ligaments that attach from the epineurium to the transverse processes and the cervical fascia sheath around the neurovascular bundle, protects the plexus from shear and tensile stresses (Fig. 1) [1,47]. Such

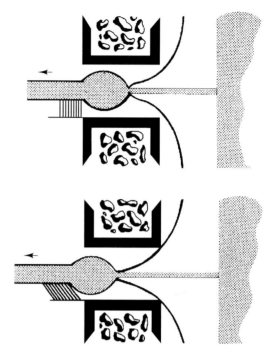

Fig. 1. Nerve roots protected from overstretch on the spinal nerve. Displacement of the nerve complex is limited by attachments of the spinal nerve to the transverse process. (*From* Sunderland S. Nerves and nerve injuries. New York: Churchill Livingstone; 1978. p. 859; with permission.)

an arrangement, together with the viscoelastic properties of peripheral nerves, minimizes the chance of a brachial plexus injury and allows for normal excursions of neck and upper-extremity movements. At the level of the clavicle, along with the axillary artery and vein, the plexus is embedded in the fascial sheath and is thus fixed to the surrounding tissues. Distally, the plexus is tethered to the surrounding tissues by its terminal branches, such as the musculocutaneous nerve, which is tethered to the coracobrachialis, the axillary nerve to the quadrilateral space, the median nerve to the pronator teres, and the ulnar nerve to the cubital sulcus.

Traction of the upper extremity in the downward direction, accompanied by flexion of the neck to the contralateral side and resulting in extreme increase in the shoulder–neck angle, can lead to injury to the upper roots and trunks. Fracture of the transverse processes can lead to disruption of root ligaments, reducing their protective function. More of the applied force is then transmitted to the roots, resulting in avulsion injury. In OBPP injuries due to shoulder dystocia, lateral traction of the head and the neck results in an increase in the shoulder–neck angle and thus in tension on the brachial plexus [48]. Forcible downward traction on the upper extremity results in an increase in the shoulder–cervical angle and injury to the upper roots and trunk. Upward traction on the arm causes widening of the scapulohumeral angle and avulsion injury to C8 and T1 roots [49]. Therefore, the magnitude of applied force and its vectors are determinants of the degree and the location of the resultant injury to the brachial plexus.

Sunderland [50] described peripheral and central mechanisms to explain injury at the roots of the brachial plexus. The term "peripheral mechanism" explains how the traction on the plexus nerves is transmitted to nerve rootlets and the dura sheath. The dura is less elastic than peripheral nerves; hence, the energy applied leads to structural failure. Within the nerve tissue, the force resulting from tensile stretch is converted to elastic potential energy and slowly retuned through viscoelastic relaxation. If excessive force is applied, the nerves give way, causing lesions to the plexus. Cervical myelography may show a pseudomeningocele. In "central mechanism," the force vectors push the cervical spine and the spinal cord to the contralateral side. These movements result in tension of the ipsilateral nerve roots. The roots rupture before the dural cones.

In general, traction forces applied to lower roots, which are unprotected by root ligaments, result in avulsion injuries. Conversely, because of the protection afforded by the root ligaments, upper roots are less susceptible to avulsion, and disruption of the upper and (to a lesser degree) the middle trunk is more common than that of the lower trunk. Clinically, this distinction is evidenced by the greater frequency of upper and middle trunk injuries compared with those of the lower trunk [1]. Furthermore, anterior rootlets are shorter and therefore more susceptible to avulsion injury than the longer posterior rootlets.

Compression injury occurs secondary to an expanding hematoma, pseudoaneurysm, and associated fracture of the clavicle. The brachial plexus may be crushed in the costovertebral space through direct trauma to the neck and the shoulders, by the direct pressure of obstetric manipulation and the use of assisting devices.

Although the brachial plexus is delicate, the undulating course of axons in the fascicles, redundancy in the surrounding epineurial and meso-neurium tissues, and the arrangement of intrinsic and extrinsic neural microvasculature allow for longitudinal excursions of peripheral nerves during limb and spine movements, without compromising structural and electrophysiologic properties of the nerve trunk.

Initial assessment

Management of infants with OBPP begins with taking a comprehensive history and performing a thorough physical examination. During physical examination, the physician can narrow down the differential diagnosis, gauge the severity of the injury, determine which nerve roots are predominantly affected, and assess the general well-being of the child.

The resting posture of the upper extremity is carefully noted. Most commonly, Erb's palsy (C5, C6 ±7) results in denervation to the deltoid, biceps, supraspinatus, teres minor, supinator, and perhaps the triceps. The resting position favors least affected muscles, and the child will hold the upper extremity in internal rotation, with adduction at the shoulder, full extension at the elbow (or slight flexion if C7 is involved), forearm in pronation, and wrist and fingers in flexion (Fig. 2). This classic posture of Erb's palsy is described as waiter's tip position [31,51,52]. Through evaluation of limb posture and affected movements, the severity of the injury and its root level can be estimated. If limb movements are weak, the child must be placed so as to eliminate gravity as a force preventing limb motion.

Assessment of associated injuries helps in further evaluation of the location and severity of brachial plexus injury. For example, abdominal asymmetry may be due to paralysis of the hemidiaphragm, which is supplied by nerve roots C3 to C5 via the phrenic

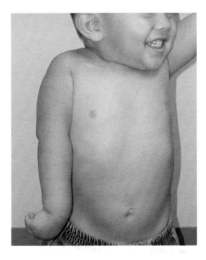

Fig. 2. Clinical presentation of Erb's palsy: shoulder in internal rotation and adduction, full extension at the elbow, forearm in pronation, wrist and fingers in flexion.

nerve, indicating that there is a high likelihood of upper root avulsions [36]. Although phrenic nerve palsy can present as an isolated lesion, it is associated with OBPP in 70% of cases [52]. Horner's syndrome is pathognomic of T1-root lesion and is most commonly associated with Klumpke's or total plexus palsy [53,54]. Cell bodies of preganglionic sympathetic neurons are located in lamina VII from T1 to L2 of the spinal cord. Preganglionic neurons pass to the paravertebral chain, which lies along the length of the vertebral column from the cervical to the sacral region. From the paravertebral chain, pre- and postganglionic neurons project to the entire

body. Normally, fibers from T1 supply head and neck structures [55]. Therefore, in total plexus or Klumpke's palsy, disruption of T1-root sympathetic fibers occurs; one manifestation of this is Horner's syndrome [32]. Sensory impairment over the neck indicates severe trauma and rupture of the cervical plexus. Assessment of the functional status of muscles innervated by nerves branching from the root (ie, long thoracic, dorsal scapular, and phrenic nerve) further helps in the diagnosis of root avulsion injuries [21,56,57]. The patient undergoes a detailed motor examination based on the Mallet and Medical Research Council Muscle Grading System motor

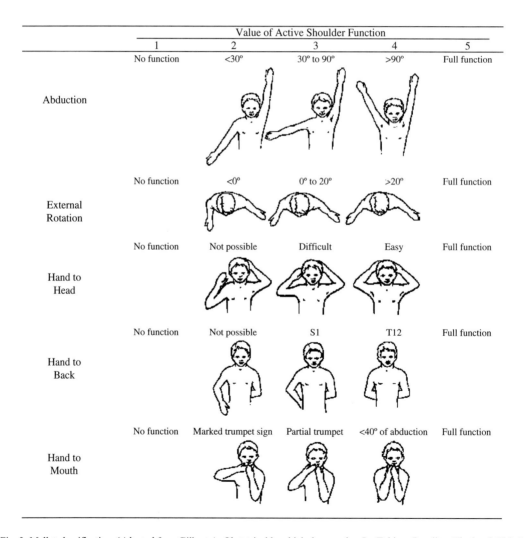

Fig. 3. Mallet classification. (*Adapted from* Gilbert A. Obstetrical brachial plexus palsy. In: Tubiana R, editor. The hand, Vol. 4. Philadelphia: WB Saunders; 1993; with permission.)

Table 1
Medical Research Council muscle grading system

Examination	Muscle grade
No contraction	0
Flicker or trace of contraction	1
Active movement, with gravity eliminated	2
Active movement against gravity	3
Active movement against gravity and resistance	4
Normal power	5

classifications to delineate the anatomic nature of the injury (Fig. 3) (Table 1).

Electrophysiologic assessment

Somatosensory evoked potentials and sensory-nerve action potentials are used to distinguish pre-ganglionic from postganglionic injuries when nerve root avulsion is suspected. When evoked potentials are created from areas of anesthesia, a preganglionic injury is assumed unless the dorsal root is also injured. Although neurophysiologic investigation is helpful in locating the position and predicting degrees of peripheral nerve injury, it has practical difficulties stemming from the intrinsic complexity of nerve interaction within the plexus and the precision of accesses due to the proximity of the overlying structures of the neck and axilla.

Intraoperatively, it is important to know if there is root avulsion; in the presence of an avulsion, an alternative donor stump will be required for neurotization of the distal stump.

Intraoperative nerve testing is done through measurement of evoked responses (in the parietal and C1 and C2 regions) by means of stimulation of exposed roots. This procedure is augmented by measurements of distal compound motor potentials through stimulation of the exposed plexus and its terminal branches. Evoked motor responses are recorded from electrodes placed on the muscles of the shoulder, arm, and hand. Intraoperative nerve testing, together with clinical examination, allows for the determination of root avulsion.

Sensory nerve action potentials (SNAPs) are used to distinguish between root avulsion and a more peripheral discontinuity, such as root rupture. Cell bodies of alpha motor neurons lie in the anterior horn of the spinal cord, where they synapse with cortico-spinal tracts and other descending pathways that modulate motor outflow. Sensory neurons have their cell bodies outside the spinal cord, in the dorsal root ganglion (DRG). Root avulsion can be differentiated based on the location of the injury with respect to DRG. A preganglionic lesion (proximal to DRG) leaves sensory neurons connected to their cell bodies while maintaining their viability and ability to conduct action potentials. However, motor neurons that are severed from their cell bodies undergo Wallerian degeneration. In a postganglionic lesion, both motor and sensory neurons undergo Wallerian degeneration.

In brachial plexus injuries occurring with concatenate root avulsions, the upper extremity movements will be affected accordingly with anesthesia in a dermatomal pattern. This result is due to the loss of central connections in both pre- and postganglionic lesions. If the limb is insensate and paretic, but SNAPs are present, this indicates root avulsion. The procedure and analysis employed with SNAPs provide a qualitative, not a quantitative assessment of presence or absence of root avulsion. Therefore, a few connecting neurons in the presence of avulsion can lead to evoked potentials and an erroneous conclusion of intact nerve roots. If there is root avulsion, distal nerve stumps will need to be neurotized to an alternative source of regenerating axons (either to other roots of the plexus or to other nerves).

Primary brachial plexus repair: rationale

Historically, OBPP was treated conservatively, because a large percentage of patients improve spontaneously and surgical intervention produced poor functional results [58,59]. Late surgical intervention produced poor results because there is a critical time period of approximately 2 years during which motor fibers must innervate the appropriate muscles—a fact not known to our predecessors. Hence, inappropriate timing of primary surgery (usually too late) coupled with poor surgical techniques yielded suboptimal functional recovery.

In general, infants have better outcomes following surgical intervention than do older patients [60]. Timing of primary surgery is critical, and, although most of the injuries improve spontaneously with good functional results, the temptation to wait is outweighed by the time constraints imposed by degenerative changes in the intramuscular nerve sheath and muscle fibers. Therefore, children who will ultimately require surgery should be treated as early as possible to optimize re-innervation of denervated muscles.

Over the years, surgeons have devised clinical algorithms to guide them in deciding whether and when surgical intervention is required. Gilbert et al [61,62] compiled characteristics that included indication for surgery if there is no biceps function at 3 months of age. However, other surgeons believe that these simple criteria can yield unacceptable false positives and that more comprehensive selection criteria are needed [31]. Hence some surgeons employ their own treatment algorithms [31,32].

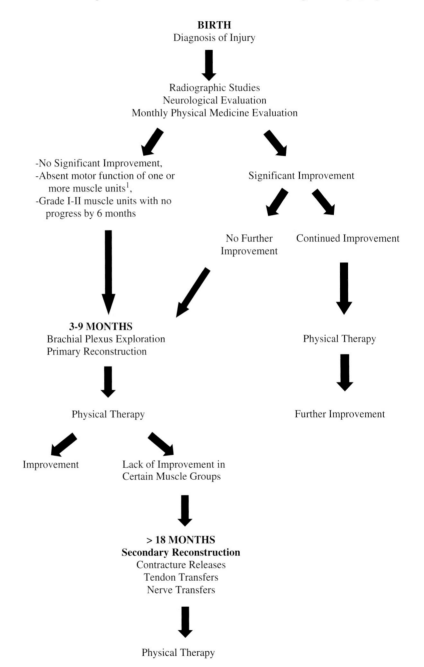

¹ elbow flexors, shoulder abductors and external rotators, and wrist and finger flexors

Fig. 4. Algorithm for treatment of obstetric brachial plexus palsy.

The authors' experience at Texas Children's Hospital has shown that, without significant deltoid, biceps, and triceps function by 3 months of life, improvement without surgical intervention is likely to yield poor results. Infants are normally operated on at the fourth month of life. Unfortunately, not all cases are seen early enough. Patients who present late may, in exceptional cases, undergo primary surgery as late as 18 months postinjury. After 12 months of age the results are disappointing. Therefore, primary reconstruction is performed when (1) total root avulsion without recovery is diagnosed by 3 months of age, (2) motor function is absent in one or more muscle units (deltoid, biceps, triceps) at 3 to 6 months of age, and (3) muscle grade I to II with no progress is seen at 6 months of age. An algorithm for timing of repair appears in Fig. 4.

In most cases, spontaneous improvement of brachial plexus injuries occurs when nerve injury is limited and the roots of the plexus are anatomically intact. Avulsed root usually leaves tufts of proximal parts attached to the spinal cord. In cases of incomplete root rupture, there may be regrowth from the proximal parts of the roots to the distal segments through the growth-supporting activity of leptomeningeal cells [63,64]. These findings indicate that under favorable conditions motor axons may be able to grow from the tufts of remnant root, along leptomeninges and the denticulate ligament, through the intervertebral canal to the distal stump [65,66]. They suggest that some degree of root-level regeneration may be taking place in patients with partial root avulsions, leading to various degrees of clinical recovery.

Primary surgery—fundamental points

Exposure of the brachial plexus is obtained by a supraclavicular incision. The roots, trunks, and early branches of the plexus are exposed above the clavicle using an incision on the posterior border of the sternocleidomastoid. The incision begins inferior to the angle of the mandible, continues inferiorly to the midportion of the clavicle, then is turned laterally toward the acromioclavicular joint. The platysma is reflected, and dissection is carried through the sternoclavicular fossa to the anterior scalene muscle. During dissection, care is taken not to damage the internal jugular vein, phrenic nerve, and the spinal accessory nerve and to preserve the cutaneous branches of the cervical plexus. At the lateral edge of the sternocleidomastoid, retraction of the omo-

hyoid assists in the identification of the phrenic nerve located on the ventral aspect of the anterior scalene muscle. Superiorly, the phrenic nerve leads to the identification of the upper roots of the plexus. The remainder of the dissection consists of exposing the plexus in an inferior lateral fashion.

At Texas Children's Hospital (TCH), the authors routinely conduct intraoperative electrophysiologic studies to facilitate clinical assessment and intraoperative findings, to assess the functional integrity of the brachial plexus, and to localize the injury as pre- or postganglionic. Once adequate operative exposure is obtained, the suspected avulsions, disruptions, and neuromas are identified for additional assessment and primary repair. Electrophysiologic assessment is performed to determine whether exposed roots are in continuity with the spinal cord. Somatic evoked potentials from stimulation of muscle groups are measured using electrodes of the parietal scalp. Nerve conduction across an area of injury including neuromas is then measured. It is the authors' practice not to excise the neuroma-incontinuity if there is less than a 50% drop in amplitude of compound motor potential across the neuroma. Microsurgical neurolysis is indicated for any neuroma that has some degree of nerve conduction (incontinuity). Intraneural compression injury from fibrosis is relieved by decompression. This measure is performed using longitudinal incisions with a 45°-angle diamond knife through the paraneurium and epineurium under 5× Loupe magnification until there is evidence of fascicular expansion. Neurolysis is performed until bands of Fontana are visible. Fasciculotomies are made to expose viable proximal and distal fascicles. This measure allows conduction to be augmented across the neuroma with fascicular grafts. Other groups who have previously performed neurolysis for conducting neuromas now prefer to excise the lesion and instead perform grafting, unless a "distinct fascicular pattern is demonstrated within the surrounding scar" [31,67]. The authors' rationale for leaving the neuroma intact is a desire not to disrupt a significant number of conducting neurons across the lesion, especially given that many of these viable neurons may be projecting through their pre-injury distal endoneurial tubes, thereby ensuring correct innervation of end organs.

If compression is still evident, continued resection of the epineurium and interfasicular exploration is performed to remove the fibrosis. If, after adequate dissection, there is still no conduction or incomplete conduction (as assessed by the degree of muscle contraction), the defect is assumed not to be incontinuity and the neuroma is excised. The proximal nerve is then resected back to normal fascicles. Viability of an avulsed nerve stump is assessed with intraoperative frozen-section analysis or by direct electrical stimulation. The presence of dorsal root ganglion cells as evidenced by frozen section or by response to stimulation excludes the possibility of avulsion. This nerve root can then be used as an intraplexal motor donor. Repair of neurotmesis or division after resection of a neuroma is facilitated by the use of nerve conduits to restore continuity and promote regeneration by direct interposition. Examples of conduits include nerve grafts, vascularized nerve grafts, veins, and synthetic bioabsorbable tubes. However, in the authors' experience, nerve grafts from the sural, great auricular, and sensory C4 nerve donors provide adequate length and the least morbidity in this population.

Cutaneous nerves are used because their removal results in minimal donor-site morbidity. Their thin trunk caliber ensures that adequate diffusion to centrally located neurons can take place, thereby diminishing the probability of central nerve trunk necrosis. The sural nerve is preferred for grafting in primary brachial plexus procedures. Because there is a possibility of a painful neuroma developing at the site where the nerve is transected, the nerve should be transected in the subfascial and not subcutaneous space [68]. Thus, even if a small-length nerve graft is used, sural nerve is harvested in its entirety. Irrespective of the conduit used, the aim of reconstruction is topographically to reunite the sensory and motor components of the nerves. Establishment of the internal orientation is accomplished with the aid of distal neurolysis and intraoperative immunohistochemical staining techniques.

When avulsion injuries are encountered, nerve transfers from functional nerve roots (neurotization) are performed to grant motor or sensory input to damaged nerves. Ruptured nerve roots provide intraplexal donors for interposition grafting to distal lesions. Extraplexal motor donors available for transfer include the phrenic, hypoglossal, and spinal accessory nerves, the motor branches of the cervical plexus, and the third through sixth intercostal nerves. Additionally, the contralateral spinal accessory nerve and the nerve roots of C7 through cross-thoracic transfer with interposition nerve grafts provide additional motor donor nerves.

Reconstruction is designed to provide maximal useful function of the limb rather than to attempt complete repair of all structures involved. Injuries resulting from complete avulsion of all the roots and multiple disruptions of the distal portions of the plexus make recovery unpredictable. Generally, re-construction should be aimed at restoration of at least two muscle groups that will provide functional ability for carrying objects, retracting the limb from danger, and stabilizing the limb. Based on these principles, restoration of muscle function should be prioritized. The highest priority is preservation of elbow flexion. Next in importance is stabilization of the shoulder—accomplished by nerve transfers to the supraspinatus and deltoid muscles. This goal is followed by reconstruction of median-innervated motor and sensory function. Because recovery of the intrinsic function of the hand is usually poor, repair of the ulnar nerve is of low priority.

The aim of the primary procedure is to restore neural connections to the denervated muscles and minimize secondary deformities. Unfortunately, a number of factors make this impossible:

- Following neuroma resection, it is not possible to guarantee correction of fascicular orientation and coaptation of proximal and distal stumps. This limitation can lead to reduction of motor and sensory innervation of appropriate end organs.
- Root avulsions mandate that donor neurons be taken from intact roots, thereby reducing quantitative innervation of the affected limb.
- Cross re-innervation may occur.
- Degenerative changes in end organs have taken place before there is significant re-innervation.

Root to plexus nerve grafting is done to avoid cross re-innervation. For example, neurotization should not involve coaptation of C6 nerve root to both the biceps and the triceps. The details of the treatment strategies are dictated by the operative findings and the time since injury; hence neurotization procedures are individualized [31]. If possible, grafting of the distal stump should be to the source route (eg, C5 and C6 to the upper trunk). If there is a root lesion or avulsion, then neurotization is done by taking fibers either from intact brachial plexus roots or from donor nerves outside the plexus. At TCH, the aims of surgery for infants and children who present with extensive brachial plexus injuries are (in order of priority) elbow flexion, shoulder abduction, external rotation, wrist extension, and finger flexion. Other centers prioritize the lower trunk for hand innervation [69,70]. However, when a significant length of time has elapsed since the injury, it may not be possible to innervate the hand in a timely manner. In these cases, grafting should focus on re-innervation of more proximal muscle groups.

The lesions that result from these brachial plexus injuries predominantly involve the upper roots.

Therefore, reconstruction is first aimed at identifying the viability of the C5, 6, and 7 roots. If the C5 root is avulsed, then the ipsilateral accessory nerve is connected to the suprascapular nerve. A neuroma of the upper trunk with intact C5 and C6 roots is corrected with multiple nerve grafts to conducting divisions. If the C7 root is damaged in this scenario, then the C6 root is joined to the middle trunk, the C5 root is attached to the upper trunk, and the suprascapular nerve is neurotized with the accessory nerve. Severe avulsions involving the entire plexus require extraplexal donors from the intercostals and the phrenic, hypoglossal, contralateral C7, and axillary nerves. Proximal donor nerve segments yield a greater number of fascicles to optimize return of function.

Thus, in a common clinical scenario, resection of an upper trunk neuroma is followed by multiple sural nerve grafts to the anterior and posterior divisions of the upper trunk and the suprascapular nerve (Fig. 5). Other surgeons prefer to graft to the level of distal cord or terminal nerve [8,71]. In a series of reconstructions for adult traumatic brachial plexus injuries, Samii et al [72] performed regression analyses of their C5-C6 nerve transfers to the musculocutaneous nerve and noted an inverse relationship between the graft length and the postoperative outcome. The authors' approach is to minimize graft length without sacrificing tension-free coaptation, appropriate donor–recipient combinations, or healthy nerve fascicles. Tension at the suture lines can lead to proliferation of scar tissue and reduction in axonal regeneration [68,73,74]. Even when the proximal and distal nerve stumps can be opposed, nerve grafting may be required to achieve tensionless repair. Table 2 outlines the reconstructive strategies

for primary repair of the brachial plexus based on the most common intraoperative presentations encountered at the authors' institution.

Terzis et al [20] published a large series of adult brachial plexus reconstructions and found that, for upper trunk lesions, intraplexal neurotizations were significantly better than extraplexal ones; for lower trunk lesions, intercostals and intraplexus nerve transfers were superior to hypoglossal and contralateral C7. For severe obstetric brachial plexus lesions where avulsions of upper roots have eliminated adequate intraplexal donors, the authors have performed a select number of cross-C7 transfers with sural nerve grafts tunneled transthoracically.

The rationale for using C7 nerve root is the abundance of myelinated axons (16,000 to 40,000) that this root contains. Theoretically, loss of C7 neural input should not lead to significant clinical limb dysfunction [75]. The sensory connections have been described as limited to the middle finger [76], or the index, middle, and ring fingers [77], or the radial side of the arm and forearm, with thumb, middle, index, and ring finger innervation [78]. In the case of multiple segmental innervations to limb muscles and extensive overlap of adjacent cutaneous innervation territories, limited sensory disruption to the skin is usually compensated by growth of neurons innervating adjacent skin regions [79]. The posterior cord receives neural contributions from all the roots of the plexus (C5–T1). This arrangement allows muscles innervated by the branches of the posterior cord to have multilevel root inputs. The central situation of C7 nerve root and the middle trunk in the brachial plexus gives us a theoretic argument for sacrificing this root, because contributions from the

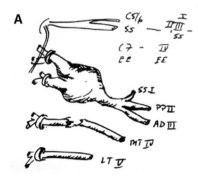
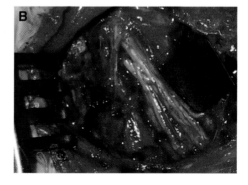

Fig. 5. (A) Intraoperative drawings demonstrating a typical lesion encountered during primary exploration. The diagram depicts a neuroma of the upper trunk and a rupture of the middle trunk. (B) Intraoperative photograph of primary brachial plexus reconstruction. After resection of a nonconducting neuroma of the upper trunk, the defect is reconstructed with multiple sural nerve grafts to the suprascapular nerve and anterior and posterior divisions.

Table 2
Strategies for primary brachial plexus reconstruction

Strategy	Injury	Reconstruction
I	Erb's Palsy	Spinal accessory nerve transfer to suprascapular nerve
	C5–C6 ruptures	C5 interpositional graft to the posterior division of the upper trunk
	C5–C6 nonconducting neuroma	C6 interpositional graft to the anterior division of the upper trunk
II	Erb's Palsy	Same as Strategy I, with C7 interpositional grafts to the middle trunk
	C5–C6 ruptures	
	C7 nonconduction Neuroma	
III	C5–T1 ruptures	Same as Strategy II, with C8 interpositional grafts to the lower trunk
IV	C5 avulsion	Spinal accessory nerve to the suprascapular nerve
	C6 rupture	C6 interpositional nerve graft to the upper trunk
V	C5–C6 ruptures	C5 interpositional nerve grafts to the suprascapular nerve and the
	C7 avulsion	posterior divisions of the upper and middle trunks
		C6 interpositional nerve grafts to the anterior division of the upper trunk
VI	Klumpke's Palsy	Partial C7 (anterior) interpositional nerve graft to the lower trunk
	C8–T1 avulsions	
VII	C5–C6 avulsions	Spinal accessory nerve transfer to suprascapular nerve
		Axillary nerve neurotization via redundant tricep branches, thoracodorsal, or subscapular nerves
		Partial ulnar nerve transfer to the musculocutaneous nerve (Oberlin procedure)
VIII	C5 rupture	C5 interpositional nerve grafts to the upper, middle, and lower trunks
	C6–T1 avulsions	
IX	Global Plexopathy	Spinal accessory nerve transfer to suprascapular nerve
	C5–T1 avulsions	Axillary nerve neurotization via multiple intercostal nerves
		Vascularized ulnar nerve graft to the median nerve
		Augmentation of reconstruction with extraplexal neurotizations (eg, hypoglossal, contralateral C7)

upper and middle trunk (through posterior divisions) should provide the affected multiroot innervated muscles with adequate numbers of functioning motor neurons. Furthermore, some motor neurons can be sacrificed because reduction in motor axons to a given muscle can lead to collateral sprouting, increasing the innervation ratio of connected motor neurons by a factor of three to five. Over time, this effect can lead to near normalization of muscle force with no obvious clinical deficits in motor function.

Following the primary procedure, it is important to minimize movement at the coaptation sites to prevent disruption of the repair and to minimize suture-site fibrosis. A brace is used to immobilize the upper limb with the shoulder in adduction and elbow flexion (at 90°) across the chest wall for approximately 4 weeks.

Correction of secondary deformities

When recovery fails following primary reconstructions or nonsurgical management, secondary deformities may arise. These deformities are a spectrum of musculoskeletal lesions, from chronic contracture to fibrosis (Table 3). Secondary procedures are necessary because of muscle imbalance, soft tissue contractures, and persistent nerve deficits that result in restricted limb function. Because of the nature of upper plexus deficits, patients are usually fixed in an internally rotated, adducted position. The adductors and the internal rotators are least affected by these deficits, whereas there is significant (or total) disruption of nerve supply to abductors and external rotators. Furthermore, gravity aids the action of adductors while hindering abduction at the shoulder joint.

Secondary reconstruction, performed at least 12 months after primary reconstruction or at 18 months of age, is designed to release the periglenoid contracture and restore abduction and external rotation with muscles transfers. Correction of most secondary defects can be accomplished with release of the subscapularis and the pectoralis at the humerus. Additionally, the axillary nerve is freed of scar by microneurolysis, followed by transfer of the

Table 3
Secondary reconstruction: indications and methods

Secondary residual deformity	Secondary quad procedure
Internal rotation	Muscle transfers to teres minor
Shoulder adduction	Latissimus dorsi
± Scapular winging	Teres major
± Biceps contracture	Muscle releases
	Subscapularis
	Pectoralis major and minor
	Axillary nerve neurolysis
	and decompression
Poor elbow extension	Nerve exploration and
	neuroplasty
	Radial nerve
	± Tendon transfers
Poor extension of wrist	Tendon transfers
and digits	PT → ECRB
Poor elbow extension	FCR → EDC
	PL →EPL
	± Wrist capsulodesis
Poor elbow flexion	Nerve exploration and
Poor supination	neuroplasty
	Radial nerve
	Musculocutaneous nerve
	± Nerve transfers
Elbow flexion contracture	Biceps lengthening after failed
	serial cast splinting
Poor flexion of wrist	Nerve exploration and
and fingers	neuroplasty
	Median nerve
	Ulnar nerve
	± Free muscle transfers

Abbreviations: ECRB, Extensor carpi radialis brevis; EDC, Extensor digitorum communis; EPL, Extensor pollicis longus; FCR, Flexor carpi radialis; PL, Palmaris longus; PT, Pronator teres.

Adapted from: Shenaq SM, et al. The surgical treatment of obstetric brachial plexus palsy. Plast Reconstr Surg 2004; 113(4):54e–67e.

teres major and latissimus dorsi to the posterior humerus to allow external rotation. Elbow flexion is restored with partial triceps transfer and lengthening. The arm is then splinted in complete abduction and external rotation for 3 months before rehabilitation begins. Although this is the most common reparative procedure, each surgical correction is tailored to the individual deficits.

Generally, secondary procedures aim to optimize limb function by facilitating shoulder abduction and external rotation and supination of the forearm. As reviewed by Jabaley [80], a number of factors related to peripheral nerve injury may explain the poor results following nerve repair. In brachial plexus injuries involving root avulsion, reduction in the total innervation of the affected limb further compounds the problem. Furthermore, out of 150,000 fibers in the brachial plexus, approximately 50,000 are required for normal shoulder function. Therefore, significant reduction in neural innervation of the upper limb can compromise the function of this joint [81].

During shoulder abduction, the torque is mainly through deltoid and supraspinatus. Infraspinatus helps beyond 120°. The muscles around the shoulder joint help to center the humeral head in the glenoid cavity during abduction at the glenohumeral joint. External rotation, by preventing impingement of the deltoid tuberosity on the coracoacromial arch, helps in abduction and also loosens the inferior glenohumeral ligaments and facilitates the positioning of the long head of the biceps centrally, allowing it to act more effectively as a humeral stabilizer. During abduction, stabilization of the humeral head against the glenoid is important. Capsulodesis of the shoulder joint is performed to optimize positioning of the head of the humerus into the glenoid cavity. Weakness of rotator cuff muscles and imbalance of forces around the shoulder joint lead to flattening of the glenoid cavity and poor development of the head of the humerus. The net result is posterior subluxation at the shoulder joint [82–85], as displayed in Fig. 6. Inferior subluxation of the shoulder joint impinges on the axillary nerve, resulting in segmental compression and further compromising abduction and external rotation. Nonabsorbable braided sutures are used to imbricate and tighten the capsule, because

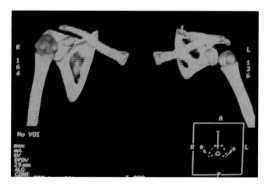

Fig. 6. Three-dimensional tomographic reconstruction of a patient with left OBPP. Skeletal deformities secondary to neuromuscular compromise of the shoulder are apparent. Note the marked humeral head hypoplasia, glenoid flattening, and posterior shoulder subluxation.

they promote scar formation through generation of local chronic inflammatory response.

Other secondary procedures consist of transferring functional muscle groups to positions that effectively restore the resultant nerve deficit. These procedures are done mostly to restore elbow flexion and external rotation of the shoulder. Transfer of the insertion of the latissimus dorsi, pectoralis major, or the triceps muscles to the biceps tendon augments flexion at the elbow. Free functional muscle grafts are used for restoration of elbow flexion and hand function. The contralateral latissimus dorsi, rectus, and gracilis are sacrificed as functional donors. Careful evaluation of motor strength and nerve conduction should be undertaken to prevent the transfer of an injured or atrophied muscle or nerve transfer from a non-conducting nerve.

Tendon transfers

Frequently, children and adults with brachial plexus lesions require tendon transfers, either because timely neural regeneration to the appropriate muscles has not taken place or because of a severe underlying injury to the plexus. Tendon transfers should be performed away from scarred tissue and skin grafts in a completely healed, nonedematous tissue. Optimal muscle force is generated at resting muscle length [86] for isometric contractions. During tendon-transfer surgery, the muscle tendon unit should therefore be transferred and sutured as close as possible to its resting length. If possible, transferred muscle should have an amplitude of excursion similar to that of the muscle whose action is being restored. It is also desirable to use a muscle tendon unit whose action is synergistic with the action being restored. Normally, some muscle or muscle groups work together to execute joint movement. An example is the synergistic action of wrist flexor and extensor muscles. Optimal grip force is exerted when the wrist is in dorsiflexion. Conversely, wrist flexion helps digit extension. When restoring wrist and digit extension, one option is to use a wrist flexor, such as flexor carpi radialis to extensor digitorum communis, palmaris longus to extensor pollicis longus, or pronator teres to extensor carpi radialis brevis [26]. For a summary of secondary procedures, see Table 3.

Nerve transfers

As a general principle, the time required for degradation of the neuromuscular endplate is approximately 18 months. After this point, nerve repair to the affected muscle group will have no benefit on rehabilitation. The sum of the time from presentation of injury and the distance the regenerating nerve has to travel (1 in per month) must be less than 18 months to allow substantial re-innervation. Strategies for overcoming this obstacle entail preserving the motor endplate through interval electric stimulation of the target muscle groups with functional nerve transfers. Nerve transfers involve connecting nerves with intact roots to distal terminal nerves close to their target muscles. This measure shortens the time to re-innervation. For example, rupture of the lateral cord will affect the musculocutaneous nerve and elbow flexion. If the thoracodorsal nerve is intact, partial transfer of its fascicles to the musculocutaneous can be performed at a location proximal to the biceps. This transfer will, in effect, decrease the denervation time of the biceps compared with a more proximal neurotization. Nerve transfers should be considered in patients who present late after injury and in patients who would be subjected to prolonged denervation intervals in primary repairs. Extreme care must be taken not to sacrifice essential functions, such as shoulder stabilization and external rotation, in donor nerve harvest.

The capacity of rerouted nerve fibers formally innervating one skeletal muscle to regenerate and innervate any other skeletal muscle has made possible nerve grafting through the denervation of muscles of a lesser function to restore more valued limb movements. Experimental evidence shows that it is the activity pattern of neural firing that induces changes in the physiologic properties of the motor units [87–90]. If possible, the donor nerve should originate from muscles with similar physiologic properties to the recipient muscles.

Long nerve grafts between the proximal and distal nerve stumps of a given nerve can lead to poor functional results. These results appear because the distance to the target muscle is too far for the axons to make contact in a timely manner before significant degenerative changes take place in muscle fibers and intramuscular nerve sheaths. It can be advantageous to use nerve transfers from nearby muscles instead of doing a primary brachial plexus repair, especially in those patients who present late after the injury. Neurotization procedures may also be required in cases of total or significant root avulsion injury of the plexus. Motor-nerve transfer is also recommended in root avulsion, when a healthy proximal stump may not be available. Neurotization may be required after primary brachial plexus surgery because of inadequate re-innervation or total denervation of a muscle.

Although a number of peripheral factors may lead to poor innervation of the end organ in brachial plexus lesions, partial avulsion of nerve roots may have occurred, which may then have coapted to distal stumps during the primary procedure. This result appears because intraoperative nerve testing does not provide a quantitative guide to the degree of connection between the roots and the spinal cord. Ultimately, insufficient numbers of motor neurons will innervate skeletal muscles, accounting for the limited return in clinical function and the need for neurotization.

The donor nerves selected have large numbers of motor axons, are in close proximity to the muscle of interest, and, if possible, innervate a muscle whose actions are synonymous with those of the muscle being innervated. Poor innervation (comparable to reduced number of axons in a donor nerve) compromises force and therefore clinical function associated with a given muscle. The distal stump (nerve to the recipient muscle) has a finite number of endoneurial tubes. Either "pure" motor nerves (such as thoracodorsal) or nerves in which motor fascicles can be readily identified (ulnar or median) should be used to ensure maximum re-innervation of the affected muscle.

Before neurotization, intraoperative nerve testing is done to assess the degree of elbow contraction. If there is inadequate or no contraction of the biceps muscle, neurotization of the biceps may be performed, provided motor axons reach the endplates within the "window of opportunity." Following a primary procedure, adequate time for nerve regeneration and innervation of the biceps muscle must be allowed before the decision is made to proceed to neurotization. If regeneration time from the plexus is deemed to be too long, significant irreversible changes in the muscle can occur.

Median and ulnar nerves supply motor axons to muscles that control wrist flexion. Moreover, wrist flexion is possible through the action of long flexors to the digits. Denervation of either flexor carpi radialis (FCR) or flexor carpi ulnaris (FCU) will not compromise wrist flexion, because the innervated muscle (either FCR or FCU) and long flexors to the hand will compensate for the weakness. The ulnar nerve has 16,000 myelinated fibers, and the median nerve has 18,000 [75]. Axons to FCR or FCU can be identified because of their large caliber and because at the level of the biceps there is good somatotopic organization within the median and ulnar nerves [91–93]. Because these nerves are close to the recipient motor endplates, interpositional nerve grafting is not required. This positioning reduces the time for

nerves to regenerate to motor endplates and reduces the number of suture sites the regenerating axons traverse. Following limited internal neurolysis of the ulnar nerve, a handheld stimulator set at 0.5 to 1 mA is used selectively to stimulate small groups of fascicles in this nerve. The aim is to use fascicles to the FCU, which are located on the lateral aspect of the ulnar nerve. At the level of the biceps, axons to FCU comprise 20% to 25% of the nerve. FCU-related fascicular stimulation will result in flexion of the wrist and ulnar deviation of the hand. No contraction of the intrinsic muscle of the hand should be seen when the fascicles to FCU are selectively stimulated. A second option is to use nerve fibers in the median nerve that supply the FCR. At the level of the biceps, neurons to FCR comprise 15% of the median nerve and are located on its superomedial aspect. If coaptation is performed between the donor nerve and the main trunk of musculocutaneous nerve, some motor fibers may grow down the lateral antebrachial-cutaneous nerve and be "wasted." It is recommended that coaptation be performed between the biceps branch of the musculocutaneous nerve and the donor nerve.

Other nerves that can be used as motor axon donors to the musculocutaneous nerve are the thoracodorsal, medial pectoral, and intercostal nerves. Following complete avulsion injury to the brachial plexus, when a primary procedure cannot be performed to restore neural input to the affected limb, one of these nerves is used for neurotization to the musculocutaneous nerve. Interpositional nerve grafting is required. Intercostal nerves have a limited number of myelinated fibers (1200–1300) compared with the musculocutaneous nerve (6000). In addition to using multiple intercostal nerves (in the form of a cable graft), one may use an intercostal nerve innervating the rectus abdominis to increase the potential motor axon count [94]. If it is anticipated that a functional muscle transfer will be required for forearm function, then neurotization may be applied to the main branch of the musculocutaneous nerve. At a later date, lateral antebrachial cutaneous nerve (LABC) may be used as a source of motor nerves to grafted functional muscle.

Physical therapy

Splinting is mandatory after secondary surgeries for two reasons. First, if sutures are used during capsulodesis, time is required for a sufficient amount of fibrous tissue to form, strengthen the capsule, and thus prevent subluxation at the glenohumeral joint.

Second, the natural tendency of the limb is adduction and internal rotation. After surgery, contractures will reform in this position, defeating the surgery's purpose. The limb is splinted in 90° abduction at the shoulder joint and full extension at the elbow joint, with the forearm in supination and external rotation at the shoulder joint. Dynamic splinting may be used in older children.

In all types of brachial plexus injury, immobility of a joint and imbalance of forces around it lead to soft tissue and muscle contractures. Loss of external rotation and abduction at the shoulder, together with contractures of the subscapularis and pectoralis major and minor, results in fixation of the limb in adduction and internal rotation. Physical and occupational therapy is instituted immediately after the injury to minimize soft tissue contractures and secondary deformities and to maintain range of joint movements. The aim is passive and, if possible, active movements of joints of the upper extremity from shoulder to finger.

Botulinum injection

In children with OBPP, biceps and triceps co-contractions can hamper or even prevent elbow flexion, leading to delayed motor development and contributing to secondary contractures and skeletal deformities. The exact mechanisms of co-contraction are unknown. It is generally believed that inappropriate rerouting of regenerating axons from the same spinal root to both the agonist and the antagonist leads to spastic co-contractions [95]. During nerve regeneration, axon collaterals from a given motor neuron have been shown to innervate functionally distinct muscles. Muscle co-contraction can occur because these sprouts are functionally competent [96].

Inappropriate co-contractions occur in children with OBPP; in persons with central nervous system disorders, co-contractions are normal during limb movements. Muscle co-contractions are defined as the simultaneous activity of agonist and antagonist muscles in the same plane on a given joint. Through in-phase firing of agonist and antagonist muscles, co-contractions increase joint stiffness; by stabilizing the joint, they help protect it from potent external forces exerted on it during physical activity and competitive sports [97]. Co-contractions increase with skill acquisition and are paramount in execution of movements that require precision and manual dexterity [98].

It has been shown clinically that botulinum toxin (BT) injection into the hyperactive antagonist (triceps) reduces co-contractions and leads to favorable long-term results in children with brachial plexus lesions. In brachial plexus palsies, two to three injections over a 12-month period have been shown to have a beneficial effect in reducing spastic co-contractions [95]. Repeated injections into the muscle do not lead to irreversible changes, induce fibrosis, or reduce the effects of subsequent injections [99]. BT injections are also used to reduce spasticity and improve resting posture in various central nervous system disorders [100–102]. BT blocks cholinergic neuromuscular transmission by inhibiting the release of acetylcholine. The electrophysiologic effects of BT outlast the clinical benefit [103].

Voluntary co-contractions involve decreased reciprocal Ia inhibition, increased presynaptic inhibition of Ia afferents, and increased Renshaw inhibition [71,104,105]. BT uptake is enhanced in the nerve terminals that are most active [106]. Following intramuscular injection, BT is also transported to ventral roots and to the adjacent spinal cord by means of retrograde axonal transport [107]. Direct stimulation of the affected muscle increases retrograde transport. In the spinal cord, BT may exert effects through various synaptic sites, including reduction in recurrent Renshaw cell inhibition [108] and reduction in the excitability of motor neurons supplying the injected muscles [109,110]. This decrease in Renshaw cell inhibition and increased presynaptic inhibition of motor neurons supplying the injected muscle may reduce spastic co-contractions [111] in central nervous system disorders. Mechanisms similar to these peripheral effects may reduce co-contractions in patients with brachial plexus lesions following muscle injections of BT.

Outcomes

At TCH, over 5000 patients with OBPP have been evaluated in the 16-year existence of the authors' program. Employing these strategies for management of OBPP, the authors have seen encouraging results. A recent review of their outcomes revealed 75% good-to-excellent (Mallet Score IV–V) results in patients who underwent primary and secondary reconstruction (n = 282). The mean follow-up interval was 5 years. This figure includes good-to-excellent outcomes in overall shoulder movement (92%), elbow flexion (86%), and hand function (62%). An

Table 4
Outcomes of brachial plexus reconstruction

	Preoperative (%)	Postoperative (%)
Primary reconstruction		
C5–C6		
Deltoid	1	26
Biceps	5	45
C5–C7		
Deltoid	0	18
Biceps	10	35
Triceps	20	57
C5–T1		
Deltoid	0	7
Biceps	0	15
Triceps	7	29
Hand	1	17

Percentage of patients with British Medical Research Council Score IV or V, with mean follow-up of 31.8 wks (n = 415).

	Preoperative (%)	Postoperative (%)
Secondary reconstruction after previous primary reconstruction (n = 58)		
Abduction > 90°	5	49
External rotation > 45°	0	36
Abduction ROM	10°	91°
External rotation ROM	0°	39°
Secondary reconstruction without previous primary reconstruction (n = 42)		
Abduction > 90°	7	59
External rotation > 45°	4	48
Abduction ROM	48°	94°
External rotation ROM	7°	46°

Mean follow-up: 1.6 y; mean age at presentation: 3.5 y; mean age at operation: 6.5 y.

Outcomes from brachial plexus reconstructions performed at Texas Children's Hospital.
Abbreviation: ROM, range of motion.

additional summary of the outcomes at TCH is outlined in Table 4.

Future directions

Re-implantation of avulsed roots

Ventral root avulsion is followed by delayed death of between 50% and 80% of motor neurons in the anterior horn of the spinal cord [64,112]. The most likely cause is not trauma due to nerve injury but severance from the peripheral nerve [64,112]. Theoretically, if original connections could be established through re-implantation of motor roots, near-normal neural input to the affected limb could be restored, obviating peripheral nerve neurotization procedures.

Investigators have shown that, following ventral root avulsion (C5–C7 injury) and reimplantation, regrowth of alpha (and, to a limited extent, gamma) motor neurons into the root occurs [113]. This regrowth takes place both with immediate and delayed (2 months postinjury) implantation [113] into the ventrolateral area of the spinal cord. Regrowth is not initiated by invasion of Schwann cells into the spinal cord; rather, regeneration is due to the activity of central nervous system–derived cells and the invasion of glial cells into the implanted root [113]. Neural connections to the implanted root are also established by neurons located on the medial aspect of the ventral horn, which is the location of cell bodies of motor neurons that innervate trunk muscles. Furthermore, co-contraction of the biceps and triceps is noted, possibly due to re-innervation of the biceps and triceps from the same motor pool. Electromyographic (EMG) evidence of re-innervation was seen within 2 to 3 months, with significant return of function within 6 to 12 months, although amplitude of the EMG was only 20% to 50% of control [114]. Although further studies are needed, experiments to date suggest the possibility of re-implanting avulsed roots into the spinal cord. However, as with peripheral nerve regeneration, selectivity may be limited, because there is evidence of cross re-innervation. This cross re-innervation may occur because motor neurons in the spinal cord are able to traverse and grow across injured areas (ie, grow to different spinal segments) [65]. The inductive influence on motor neural growth (neurotropic factors and local disruption in the blood–brain barrier) [115] is generalized at least across the adjacent segments of the spinal cord, resulting in spinal connections to inappropriate nerve roots. As with peripheral nerve regeneration following nerve repair, re-innervation selectivity may thus be limited. During peripheral nerve regeneration, axonal pruning associated with remodeling of regenerating neurons increases the precision of organ re-innervation [116]. It is therefore not unreasonable to assume that similar processes may occur following ventral root implantation.

Bionics

Following functional muscle transfer, 12 to 18 months may elapse before clinical evidence of voluntary muscle contraction appears. In the interim, degenerative changes take place in the grafted muscle. Therefore, it may be beneficial to use cuff electrodes (or their equivalent) and record mass activity from the donor nerve to the grafted muscle. Recorded, amplified, filtered motor neural signals could then be channeled to the grafted muscle by means of intramuscular electrodes. Alternatively, surface electrodes could be used. This procedure will hinder muscle atrophy, and it is to be hoped that, soon after the muscle transfer procedure, the permissive effect of joint movement will stimulate patient cooperation with further rehabilitation therapy.

Stem cells

Tissues consist of two basic cell types, postmitotic cells and stem cells. The former are responsible for maintaining physiologic activities, and the latter are responsible for replenishing the postmitotic cell during times of tissue injury or growth. As an organism matures from an embryo to an adult, the number of postmitotic cells increases and the population of stem cells declines; in some tissues there is complete depletion of stem cell numbers. Properties that define stem cells include undifferentiation, capability of proliferation and self-renewal, ability to produce large numbers of differentiated progeny, and regeneration potential after tissue injury [117]. Stem cells change their phenotype according to their local microenvironment, which is a conglomerate of locally secreted factors and extracellular matrix [118–121], with physiologic effects mediated by complex interactions through a multitude of growth and regulatory factors [122–124]. In experimental models, incorporation of Schwann cells into biologic nerve conduits has been shown to enhance nerve regeneration. Not only are human Schwann cells technically difficult to purify, but culture and clonal proliferation are time-consuming, with a lag time of up to 10 weeks [125]. A possible solution is to use stem cells. Although Schwann progenitor cells have been identified in rat fetal sciatic nerve [126], there is no evidence that stem cells exist in adult peripheral nervous tissues. As an alternative, possible candidate cells for transplantation into conduits include neural progenitor cells, olfactory ensheathing cells, and mesenchymal stem cell–derived cells.

Summary

Management of brachial plexus injuries is geared toward normalization of limb function, primarily through optimization of nerve regeneration and mechanical increase in elbow flexion and shoulder stabilization. Changes in the skeletal muscles and the osteous structures of the upper extremity are ongoing throughout the course of treatment, mandating continual assessment and aggressive rehabilitation. In patients who present too late for microsurgical intervention, irreversible changes take place in skeletal muscles, highlighting the importance of early referral. However, secondary procedures have been shown to be beneficial in older patients and in those whose primary procedures failed. Further advances in bionics and stem cell therapy may help replace the dynamic functional deficits of OBPP.

Acknowledgments

The authors would like to thank all the members of the Brachial Plexus Team at Texas Children's Hospital:
Aloysia Schwabe, MD—Physical Rehabilitation and Physical Medicine Rehabilitation Clinic
Lisa Davis, RN—Clinic/Nurse Coordinator
Gail Fuller—Clinic/Nurse Coordinator
Lisa Thompson—Clinic Coordinator
Angel Gonzales—Clinic Coordinator
Nancy Conte—Occupational Therapist
Cheryl Mitchell—Occupational Therapist
Jeanie Murphy—Occupational Therapist
Rose Banda—Occupational Therapist

References

[1] Sunderland S. Nerves and nerve injuries. New York: Churchill Livingstone; 1978.
[2] Leon SFE. The first reported case of radial nerve palsy. South Med J 1993;86:808–11.
[3] Awad IA. Galen's anecdote of the fallen sophist: on the certainty of science through anatomy. J Neurosurg 1995;83(5):929–32.
[4] Shenaq SM, Kim JY, Armenta AH, Nath RK, Cheng E, Jedrysiak A. The surgical treatment of obstetric brachial plexus palsy. Plast Reconstr Surg 2004; 113(4):54e–67e.
[5] Leffert RD. Brachial plexus injuries. New York: Churchill Livingstone; 1985.
[6] Duchenne GBA. De l'electrization localisée et de son application à la pathologie et à la thérapeutique. 3rd edition. Paris: Balliere; 1872.
[7] Erb W. Uber eine eigenthumliche Localisation von Lahmungen in Plexus brachialis. Verhandlungen Naturkinde Medizin 1874;2:130–1.
[8] Klumpke A. Contribution à l'étude des paralysies radiculaires du plexus brachial: paralysies radiculaires totales: paralysies radicularies inférieures: de la participation des filets sympathiques oculo-pupillaires dans ces paralysies. Rev Med Suisse Romande 1885; 5:591–616.
[9] Seeligmuller ID. Brachial plexus. Dtsch Arch Klin Med 1877;20:101–3.

[10] Terzis JK, Papakonstantinou KC. The surgical treatment of brachial plexus injuries in adults. Plast Reconstr Surg 2000;106:1097–112.

[11] Taylor AS. Brachial birth palsy and injuries of similar type in adults. Surg Gynecol Obstet 1920;30: 494–502.

[12] Wyeth JA, Sharp W. The field of neurological surgery in a general hospital. Surg Gynecol Obstet 1917; 24:29–36.

[13] Seddon HJ. The use of autogenous grafts for the repair of large gaps in peripheral nerves. Br J Surg 1947;35:151–66.

[14] Leffert RD. Brachial-plexus injuries. N Engl J Med 1974;29:1059–67.

[15] Narakas A. Surgical treatment of traction injuries of the brachial plexus. Clin Orthop 1978;133:71–90.

[16] Narakas AO. The surgical treatment of traumatic brachial plexus lesions. Int Surg 1980;65(6):521–7.

[17] Millesi H. Surgical management of brachial plexus injuries. J Hand Surg [Am] 1977;2:367–78.

[18] Millesi H. Brachial plexus injury in adults: operative repair. In: Gelberman RH, editor. Operative nerve repair and reconstruction. Philadelphia: JP Lippincott; 1991. p. 1285–301.

[19] Terzis JK. Brachial plexus reconstruction in 204 patients with devastating paralysis. Plast Reconstr Surg 1999;104:1221–40.

[20] Terzis JK, Liberson WT, Levine R. Obstetric brachial plexus palsy. Hand Clin 1986;2:773–86.

[21] Tung TH, Mackinnon SE. Brachial plexus injuries. Clin Plast Surg 2003;30(2):269–87.

[22] Gilbert A, Hentz VR, Tassin JL. Brachial plexus reconstruction in obstetrical palsy: operative indications and postoperative results. In: Urbaniak JR, editor. Microsurgery for major limb reconstruction. St. Louis (MO): CV Mosby; 1987. p. 348–64.

[23] Gilbert A. Long-term evaluation of brachial plexus surgery in obstetrical palsy. Hand Clin 1995;11: 583–94 [discussion: 594–5].

[24] Gilbert A, Khouri N, Carlioz H. Birth palsy of the brachial plexus: surgical exploration and attempted repair in twenty-one cases. Rev Chir Orthop Reparatrice Appar Mot 1980;66(1):33–42.

[25] Boome RS, Kaye JC. Obstetric traction injuries of the brachial plexus: natural history, indications for surgical repair and results. J Bone Joint Surg Br 1988; 70:571–6.

[26] Shenaq SM, Berzin E, Lee R, Laurent JP, Nath R, Nelson MR. Brachial plexus birth injuries and current management. Clin Plast Surg 1998;25:527–36.

[27] Shenaq SM. Obstetrical brachial plexus palsy: a twelve-year experience with 1012 cases. Presented at American Society for Reconstructive Microsurgery. Hawaii, January 12–20, 1999.

[28] Laurent JP, Lee R, Shenaq S, Parke JT, Solis IS, Kowalik L. Neurosurgical correction of upper brachial plexus birth injuries. J Neurosurg 1993;79:197–203.

[29] Laurent JP, Lee RT. Birth-related upper brachial plexus injuries in infants: operative and nonoperative approaches. J Child Neurol 1994;9:111–7 [discussion: 118].

[30] Wei JN, Wang SH, Liu SF. [Peripheral nerve repair of the upper limb: an analysis of 87 cases.] Chung Hua Wai Ko Tsa Chih 1981;19(1):3–6.

[31] Marcus JR, Clarke HM. Management of obstetrical brachial plexus palsy evaluation, prognosis, and primary surgical treatment. Clin Plast Surg 2003;30: 289–306.

[32] Michelow BJ, Clarke HM, Curtis CG, Zuker RM, Seifu Y, Andrews DF. The natural history of obstetrical brachial plexus palsy. Plast Reconstr Surg 1994;94:675–80.

[33] Levine MG, Holroyde J, Woods Jr JR, Siddiqu TA, Scott M, Miodovnik M. Birth trauma: incidence and predisposing factors. Obstet Gynecol 1984;63: 792–5.

[34] Hardy AE. Birth injuries of the brachial plexus: incidence and prognosis. J Bone Joint Surg Br 1981; 63B:98–101.

[35] Gilbert A, Nesbitt TS, Danielsen B. Associated factors in 1611 cases of brachial plexus injury. Obstet Gynecol 1999;93:536–40.

[36] Al Qattan MM, Clarke HM, Curtis CG. The prognostic value of concurrent phrenic nerve palsy in newborn children with Erb's palsy. J Hand Surg [Br] 1998;23:225.

[37] Specht EE. Brachial plexus palsy in the newborn: incidence and prognosis. Clin Orthop 1975;110:32–4.

[38] Eng GD, Koch B, Smokuyina MD. Brachial plexus palsy in neonates and children. Arch Phys Med Rehabil 1978;59:458–64.

[39] Jennett RJ, Tarby TJ. Brachial plexus palsy: an old problem revisited again. II. Cases in point. Am J Obstet Gynecol 1997;176:1356–7.

[40] Jennett RJ, Tarby TJ, Kreinick CJ. Brachial plexus palsy: an old problem revisited. Am J Obstet Gynecol 1992;166:1673–7.

[41] Sjoberg I, Erichs K, Bjerre I. Cause and effect of obstetric (neonatal) brachial plexus palsy. Acta Paediatr Scand 1988;77:357–64.

[42] Hentz VR, Meyer RD. Brachial plexus microsurgery in children. Microsurgery 1991;12:175–85.

[43] Brown KL. Review of obstetrical palsies: nonoperative treatment. Clin Plast Surg 1984;11:181–7.

[44] Metaizeau JP, Gayet C, Plenat F. Brachial plexus birth injuries: an experimental study. Chir Pediatr 1979; 20(3):159–63.

[45] Metaizeau JP, Prevot J, Lascombes P. Obstetrical paralysis: spontaneous development and results of early microsurgical treatment. Ann Pediatr (Paris) 1984;31(2):93–102.

[46] Geutjens G, Gilbert A, Helsen K. Obstetric brachial plexus palsy associated with breech delivery: a different pattern of injury. J Bone Joint Surg Br 1996; 8:303–6.

[47] Mansat M. [Surgical topographic anatomy of the brachial plexus.] Rev Chir Orthop Reparatrice Appar Mot 1977;63:20–6.

[48] Clarke HM, Curtis CG. An approach to obstetrical brachial plexus injuries. Hand Clin 1995;11:563–80 [discussion: 580–1].

[49] Coene LN. Mechanisms of brachial plexus lesions. Clin Neurol Neurosurg 1993;95(Suppl):S24–9.

[50] Sunderland S. Mechanisms of cervical nerve root avulsion in injuries of the neck and shoulder. J Neurosurg 1974;41:705–14.

[51] Brown KL. Review of obstetrical palsies. Nonoperative treatment. Clin Plast Surg 1984;11:181–7.

[52] Slooff AC. Obstetric brachial plexus lesions and their neurosurgical treatment. Microsurgery 1995;16: 30–4.

[53] Jennett RJ, Tarby TJ, Krauss RL. Erb's palsy contrasted with Klumpke's and total palsy: different mechanisms are involved. Am J Obstet Gynecol 2002;186:1216–9 [discussion: 1219–20].

[54] Al-Qattan MM, Clarke MH, Curtis CG. The prognostic value of concurrent Horner's syndrome in total obstetric brachial plexus injury. J Hand Surg [Br] 2000;25:166–7.

[55] Martini FH, Tommons MJ, Tallitsch RB. Human anatomy. Reason Benjamin Cummings 2002;89.

[56] Alnot JY. Traumatic brachial plexus lesions in the adult. Indications and results. Hand Clin 1995;11: 623–31.

[57] Balakrishnan G, Kadadi BK. Clinical examination versus routine and paraspinal electromyographic studies in predicting the site of lesion in brachial plexus injury. J Hand Surg [Am] 2004;29:140–3.

[58] Robotti E, Longhi P, Verna G, Bocchiotti G. Brachial plexus surgery. An historical perspective. Hand Clin 1995;11:517–33.

[59] Duclos L, Gilbert A. Obstetrical palsy: early treatment and secondary procedures. Ann Acad Med Singapore 1995;24:841–5.

[60] Hentz VR, Narakas A. The results of microneurosurgical reconstruction in complete brachial plexus palsy. Assessing outcome and predicting results. Orthop Clin North Am 1988;19:107–14.

[61] Gilbert A, Razaboni R, Amar-Khodja S. Indications and results of brachial plexus surgery in obstetrical palsy. Orthop Clin North Am 1988;19:91–105.

[62] Gilbert A, Brockman R, Carlioz H. Surgical treatment of brachial plexus birth palsy. Clin Orthop 1991; 264:39–47.

[63] Risling M, Dalsgaard CJ, Terenius L. Neuropeptide Y-like immunoreactivity in the lumbosacral pia mater in normal cats and after sciatic neuroma formation. Brain Res 1985;358:372–5.

[64] Risling M, Fried K, Linda H, Carlstedt T, Cullheim S. Regrowth of motor axons following spinal cord lesions: distribution of laminin and collagen in the CNS scar tissue. Brain Res Bull 1993;30:405–14.

[65] Risling M, Aldskogius H, Hildebrand C, Remahl S. Effects of sciatic nerve resection on L7 spinal roots and dorsal root ganglia in adult cats. Exp Neurol 1983;82:568–80.

[66] Smith KJ, Kodama T. Reinnervation of denervated skeletal muscle by central neurons regenerating via ventral roots implanted into the spinal cord. Brain Res 1991;551:221–9.

[67] Clarke HM, Al-Qattan MM, Curtis CG, Zuker RM. Obstetrical brachial plexus palsy: results following neurolysis of conducting neuromas-in-continuity. Plast Reconstr Surg 1996;97:974–82 [discussion: 983–4].

[68] Millesi H. Techniques for nerve grafting. Hand Clin 2000;16:73–91,viii.

[69] Borrero JL. Surgical technique. In: Gilbert A, editor. Brachial plexus injuries. London: Martin Dunitz; 2001. p. 205–10.

[70] Gilbert A. Indications and strategy. In: Gilbert A, editor. Brachial plexus injuries. London: Martin Dunitz; 2001. p. 198–204.

[71] Nielsen J, Kagamihara Y. The regulation of presynaptic inhibition during co-contraction of antagonistic muscles in man. J Physiol 1993;464:575–93.

[72] Samii M, Carvalho GA, Nikkhah G, Penkert G. Surgical reconstruction of the musculocutaneous nerve in traumatic brachial plexus injuries. J Neurosurg 1997;87:881–6.

[73] Millesi H. Healing of nerves. Clin Plast Surg 1977; 4:459–73.

[74] Millesi H, Meissl G, Berger A. Further experience with interfascicular grafting of the median, ulnar, and radial nerves. J Bone Joint Surg Am 1976;58: 209–18.

[75] Narakas AO. Thoughts on neurotization or nerve transfers in irreparable nerve lesions. Clin Plast Surg 1984;11:153–9.

[76] Narakas A. Brachial plexus surgery. Orthop Clin North Am 1981;12:303–23.

[77] Carpenter MB. Human neuroanatomy. Baltimore (MD): Williams & Wilkins; 1976.

[78] Last RJ. Anatomy: regional and applied. New York: Churchill Livingstone; 1977.

[79] Bishop B. Neural plasticity: Part 3. Responses to lesions in the peripheral nervous system. Phys Ther 1982;62:1275–82.

[80] Jabaley ME. Technical aspects of peripheral nerve repair. J Hand Surg [Br] 1984;9(1):14–9.

[81] Allieu Y, Cenac P. Is surgical intervention justifiable for total paralysis secondary to multiple avulsion injuries of the brachial plexus? Hand Clin 1988;4: 609–18.

[82] Waters PM, Smith GR, Jaramillo D. Glenohumeral deformity secondary to brachial plexus birth palsy. J Bone Joint Surg Am 1998;80:668–77.

[83] Pearl ML, Edgerton BW. Glenoid deformity secondary to brachial plexus birth palsy. J Bone Joint Surg Am 1998;80:659–67.

[84] Dunkerton MC. Posterior dislocation of the shoulder associated with obstetric brachial plexus palsy. J Bone Joint Surg Br 1989;71:764–6.

[85] Beischer AD, Simmons TD, Torode IP. Glenoid version in children with obstetric brachial plexus palsy. J Pediatr Orthop 1999;19:359–61.

[86] Liebrer RL. Skeletal muscle structure, function and plasticity. 2nd edition. Philadelphia: Lippincott Williams & Wilkins; 2002.

[87] Eken T, Gundersen K. Electrical stimulation resembling normal motor-unit activity: effects on denervated fast and slow rat muscles. J Physiol 1988; 402:651–69.

[88] Eerbeek O, Kernell D, Verhey BA. Effects of fast and slow patterns of tonic long-term stimulation on contractile properties of fast muscle in the cat. J Physiol 1984;352:73–90.

[89] Salmons S, Vrbova G. The influence of activity on some contractile characteristics of mammalian fast and slow muscles. J Physiol 1969;201:535–49.

[90] Salmons S, Sreter FA. Significance of impulse activity in the transformation of skeletal muscle type. Nature 1976;263:30–4.

[91] Ekedahl R, Frank O, Hallin RG. Peripheral afferents with common function cluster in the median nerve and somatotopically innervate the human palm. Brain Res Bull 1997;42:367–76.

[92] Hallin RG. Microneurography in relation to intraneural topography: somatotopic organisation of median nerve fascicles in humans. J Neurol Neurosurg Psychiatry 1990;53:736–44.

[93] Schady W, Ochoa JL, Torebjork HE, Chen LS. Peripheral projections of fascicles in the human median nerve. Brain 1983;106:745–60.

[94] Highet WB, Saunders FK. The effect of stretching nerves after suture. Br J Surg 1943;30:355–71.

[95] Rollnik JD, Hierner R, Schubert M, Shen ZL, Johannes S, Troger M, et al. Botulinum toxin treatment of cocontractions after birth-related brachial plexus lesions. Neurology 2000;55:112–4.

[96] Esslen E. Electromyographic findings on two types of misdirection of regenerating axons. Electroencephalogr Clin Neurophysiol 1960;12:738–41.

[97] Hagood S, Solomonow M, Baratta R, Zhou BH, D'Ambrosia R. The effect of joint velocity on the contribution of the antagonist musculature to knee stiffness and laxity. Am J Sports Med 1990;18:182–7.

[98] Humphrey DR, Reed DJ. Separate cortical systems for control of joint movement and joint stiffness: reciprocal activation and coactivation of antagonist muscles. Adv Neurol 1983;39:347–72.

[99] Sloop RR, Cole D, Patel MC. Muscle paralysis produced by botulinum toxin type A injection in treated torticollis patients compared with toxin naive individuals. Mov Disord 2001;16:100–5.

[100] Rodriquez AA, McGinn M, Chappell R. Botulinum toxin injection of spastic finger flexors in hemiplegic patients. Am J Phys Med Rehabil 2000;79:44–7.

[101] Dunne JW, Heye N, Dunne SL. Treatment of chronic limb spasticity with botulinum toxin A. J Neurol Neurosurg Psychiatry 1995;58:232–5.

[102] Corry IS, Cosgrove AP, Walsh EG, McClean D, Graham HK. Botulinum toxin A in the hemiplegic upper limb: a double-blind trial. Dev Med Child Neurol 1997;39:185–93.

[103] Odergren T, Hjaltason H, Kaakkola S, Solders G, Hanko J, Fehling C, et al. A double blind, randomised, parallel group study to investigate the dose equivalence of Dysport and Botox in the treatment of cervical dystonia. J Neurol Neurosurg Psychiatry 1998;64:6–12.

[104] Nielsen J, Sinkjaer T, Toft E, Kagamihara Y. Segmental reflexes and ankle joint stiffness during co-contraction of antagonistic ankle muscles in man. Exp Brain Res 1994;102:350–8.

[105] Nielsen J, Kagamihara Y. The regulation of disynaptic reciprocal Ia inhibition during co-contraction of antagonistic muscles in man. J Physiol 1992;456: 373–91.

[106] Hughes R, Whaler BC. Influence of nerve-ending activity and of drugs on the rate of paralysis of rat diaphragm preparations by Cl. botulinum type A toxin. J Physiol 1962;160:221–33.

[107] Boroff DA, Chen GS. On the question of permeability of the blood–brain barrier to botulinum toxin. Int Arch Allergy Appl Immunol 1975;48: 495–504.

[108] Hamjian JA, Walker FO. Serial neurophysiological studies of intramuscular botulinum-A toxin in humans. Muscle Nerve 1994;17:1385–92.

[109] Pauri F, Boffa L, Cassetta E, Pasqualetti P, Rossini PM. Botulinum toxin type-A treatment in spastic paraparesis: a neurophysiological study. J Neurol Sci 2000;181:89–97.

[110] Pauri F, Boffa L, Cassetta E, Pasqualetti P, Rossini PM. Botulinum toxin type-A treatment in spasticity increases the central conduction time to brain stimulation. Electroencephalogr Clin Neurophysiol Suppl 1999;51:250–9.

[111] Hultborn H, Jankowska E, Lindstrom S. Recurrent inhibition from motor axon collaterals of transmission in the Ia inhibitory pathway to motoneurones. J Physiol 1971;215:591–612.

[112] Hoffmann CF, Thomeer RT, Marani E. Reimplantation of ventral rootlets into the cervical spinal cord after their avulsion: an anterior surgical approach. Clin Neurol Neurosurg 1993;95(Suppl):S112–8.

[113] Cullheim S, Carlstedt T, Linda H, Risling M, Ulfhake B. Motoneurons reinnervate skeletal muscle after ventral root implantation into the spinal cord of the cat. Neuroscience 1989;29:725–33.

[114] Carlstedt TP, Hallin RG, Hedstrom KG, Nilsson-Remahl IA. Functional recovery in primates with brachial plexus injury after spinal cord implantation of avulsed ventral roots. J Neurol Neurosurg Psychiatry 1993;56:649–54.

[115] Yan Q, Elliott J, Snider WD. Brain-derived neurotrophic factor rescues spinal motor neurons from axotomy-induced cell death. Nature 1992;360:753–5.

[116] Bennett M, Ho S, Lavidis N. Competition between segmental nerves at end-plates in rat gastrocnemius muscle during loss of polyneuronal innervation. J Physiol 1986;381:351–76.

[117] Potten CS, Loeffler M. Stem cells: attributes, cycles,

spirals, pitfalls and uncertainties. Lessons for and from the crypt. Development 1990;110:1001–20.

[118] Ginis I, Rao MS. Toward cell replacement therapy: promises and caveats. Exp Neurol 2003;184:61–77.

[119] Fuchs E, Segre JA. Stem cells: a new lease on life. Cell 2000;100:143–55.

[120] Shah NM, Groves AK, Anderson DJ. Alternative neural crest cell fates are instructively promoted by TGFbeta superfamily members. Cell 1996;85: 331–43.

[121] Shah NM, Marchionni MA, Isaacs I, Stroobant P, Anderson DJ. Glial growth factor restricts mammalian neural crest stem cells to a glial fate. Cell 1994; 77:349–60.

[122] Estes BT, Gimble JM, Guilak F. Mechanical signals as regulators of stem cell fate. Curr Top Dev Biol 2004;60:91–126.

[123] Verfaillie CM, McCarthy JB, McGlave PB. Differentiation of primitive human multipotent hematopoietic progenitors into single lineage clonogenic progenitors is accompanied by alterations in their interaction with fibronectin. J Exp Med 1991;174: 693–703.

[124] Gronthos S, Simmons PJ. The growth factor requirements of STRO-1–positive human bone marrow stromal precursors under serum-deprived conditions in vitro. Blood 1995;85:929–40.

[125] Zandstra PW, Nagy A. Stem cell bioengineering. Annu Rev Biomed Eng 2001;3:275–305.

[126] Mosahebi A, Woodward B, Wiberg M, Martin R, Terenghi G. Retroviral labeling of Schwann cells: in vitro characterization and in vivo transplantation to improve peripheral nerve regeneration. Glia 2001; 34:8–17.

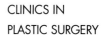

CLINICS IN
PLASTIC SURGERY

**ELSEVIER
SAUNDERS**

Clin Plastic Surg 32 (2005) 99 – 116

Current management of hemangiomas and vascular malformations

Jennifer J. Marler, MD[a],*, John B. Mulliken, MD[b]

[a]Division of Plastic Surgery, Department of Surgery, Cincinnati Children's Medical Center, ML2020, 3333 Burnet Avenue,
Cincinnati, OH 45229, USA
[b]Division of Plastic Surgery, Department of Surgery, Children's Hospital and Harvard Medical School, Hunnewell 178,
300 Longwood Avenue, Boston, MA 02115, USA

Vascular anomalies is a new, rapidly evolving multidisciplinary field that combines several surgical and medical specialities. The plastic surgeon plays an essential role in the management of affected patients.

The greatest impediment to development of this field has been confusing terminology. This has been responsible for improper diagnosis, illogical treatment, and misdirected research. However, a biologic classification system introduced in 1982 based on studies correlating physical findings, natural history, and cellular features has clarified most of this terminologic disorder [1]. There are two major categories of vascular anomalies: tumors and malformations (Box 1).

Vascular tumors are endothelial neoplasms characterized by increased cellular proliferation. Hemangioma is the most common and is almost exclusive to infants. Other tumors are hemangioendotheliomas, tufted angioma, hemangiopericytomas, and other rare vascular neoplasms, including angiosarcoma. Vascular malformations, on the other hand, are the result of abnormal development of vascular elements during embryogenesis and fetal life. These may be single vessel forms (capillary, arterial, lymphatic, or venous) or a combination. Vascular malformations do not generally demonstrate increased endothelial turnover. They are designated according to the predominant channel type as capillary malformations, lymphatic malformations, venous malformations, arteriovenous malformations, and complex forms such as capillary-

lymphatico-venous malformation. Malformations with an arterial component are rheologically fast-flow, while the remainder are slow-flow.

There are rare exceptions to this classification scheme. Vascular malformations, while essentially structural disorders, can demonstrate endothelial hyperplasia, possibly triggered by clotting, ischemia, embolization, partial resection, or hormonal influences. Rarely, vascular tumors and vascular malformations can coexist. For example, pyogenic granuloma, a tiny acquired vascular tumor, often appears in the dermis along with a capillary malformation.

History and physical examination can distinguish between vascular tumors and vascular malformations with a diagnostic accuracy of over 90% [2]. The most common error in determining a clinical diagnosis continues to be the inaccurate and imprecise use of terminology. Perhaps the most extreme example is the term *hemangioma*, which is frequently applied generically and indiscriminately to vascular lesions that are entirely different in histology and behavior. *Cavernous hemangioma* is a similar offender, because in reality there is no such entity—a lesion is either a deep hemangioma or a venous malformation.

Vascular tumors

Hemangioma

Pathogenesis

Hemangiomas are endothelial tumors with a unique biologic behavior—they grow rapidly, regress

* Corresponding author.
E-mail address: jennifer.marler@cchmc.org (J.J. Marler).

0094-1298/05/$ – see front matter © 2005 Elsevier Inc. All rights reserved.
doi:10.1016/j.cps.2004.10.001

plasticsurgery.theclinics.com

Box 1. Vascular anomalies

Tumors

    Hemangioma
    Pyogenic granuloma
    Kaposiform hemangioendothelioma
    Other rare tumors

Malformations

    Capillary
    Lymphatic
    Venous
    Arteriovenous
    Combined

slowly, and never recur. The three stages in the life cycle of a hemangioma, each characterized by a unique assemblage of biologic markers and processes, are (1) the proliferating phase (0–1 year of age), (2) the involuting phase (1–5 years of age), and (3) the involuted phase (>5 years of age). These stages are typically clinically apparent and can be distinguished microscopically and immunohistochemically [3].

In the proliferating phase, the hemangioma is composed of plump, rapidly dividing endothelial cells that form tightly packed sinusoidal channels. Even at this early stage, the endothelial cells express phenotypic markers of mature endothelium [3], in addition to markers of activated endothelium. Urinary markers of angiogenesis, such as basic fibroblast growth factor and high molecular weight (MW) matrix metalloproteinases (MMPs) are usually high in infants with proliferating hemangiomas and diminish to normal levels during regression [4,5]. In the involuting phase, there is decreasing endothelial proliferation, increasing apoptosis, and the beginning of fibrofatty replacement of the hemangioma. The net result is loss of volume of the tumor and increasing softness of the overlying skin. During the involuted phase, after regression is complete, all that remains are a few tiny capillary-like feeding vessels and draining veins (some of which can be abnormally large) surrounded by islands of fibrofatty tissue admixed with dense collagen and reticular fibers. The endothelium lining these vessels is flat and mature. Multilaminated basement membranes persist around the residual tiny capillary-sized vessels.

Clinical features

Hemangioma is the most common tumor of infancy and childhood, occurring in 4% to 10% of Caucasian infants. These lesions are three to five times more common in females, with an even higher female preponderance in hemangiomas that are problematic or associated with structural abnormalities. There is an increased frequency of hemangiomas in premature infants with a reported incidence of 23% in neonates who weigh less than 1200 g [6]. Hemangiomas are unusual in dark-skinned infants.

Hemangiomas are generally noted within the first 2 weeks of postnatal life. However, there is wide variability in this timing. Deep subcutaneous lesions, such as in the parotid, may not be noted by until the infant is several months old. Their appearance is heralded, in 30% to 50% of infants, by a premonitory cutaneous mark that may resemble a pale spot, telangiectatic or macular red stain, or a bruise-like pseudoecchymotic patch. Hemangiomas occur most commonly in the craniofacial region (60%), followed by the trunk (25%) and extremities (15%) [2]. Eighty percent of cutaneous hemangiomas are single, while 20% are multiple. Multiple cutaneous lesions often are associated with hemangiomas in other organ systems, particularly the liver.

The presentation of hemangiomas is variable in terms of size, extent and morphology (Fig. 1). When there is superficial dermal involvement, the skin becomes raised, firm and bosselated with a vivid crimson color. If the hemangioma is limited to the deeper dermis, subcutaneous tissue or muscle, the overlying skin may be only slightly raised, warm, and have a bluish hue. All of these structures may be involved with a superficial raised component overlying a deeper tumor. Hemangioma in an extremity may present with a macular, telangiectatic appearance. The adjectives *cavernous* and *capillary*— previously used to describe deep and superficial hemangiomas, respectively—are confusing and inaccurate and should thus be eliminated [1,7].

The three stages of histologic appearance of hemangioma correlate with its clinical course [1]. During the proliferating phase, growth is rapid and frequent observation is needed to document the growth pattern. Few indicators predict the eventual volume of a particular hemangioma or forecast the timing and outcome of involution. Typically, hemangiomas begin to plateau in growth by 10 to 12 months, although some demonstrate growth stabilization earlier or later.

During the involuting phase, after 1 year of age, the growth of the hemangioma slows, and, for a time, is commensurate to that of the child. The

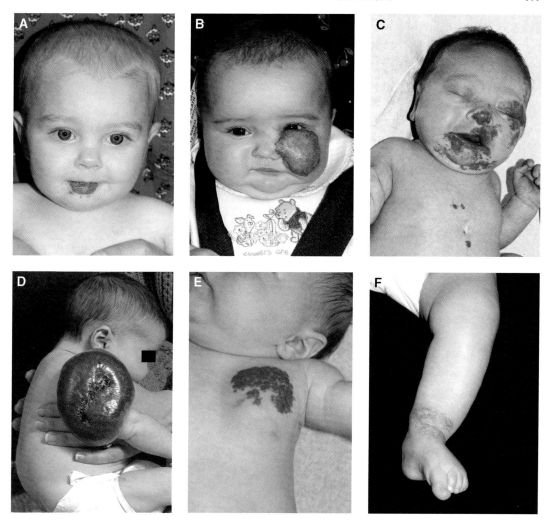

Fig. 1. Variable morphologic appearances of hemangioma, illustrated in patients (*A–F*). Patient C has associated PHACES syndrome with carotid and aortic arch abnormalities. Note the sternal cleft.

telltale signs of regression appear. The skin begins to pale, typically beginning at the center of the lesion and a patchy grayish discoloration becomes discernable. The hemangioma is softer on palpation. The involuting phase extends from 1 year until 5 to 7 years of age. The rate of regression is unrelated to the appearance, depth, gender, site, or size of the hemangioma [2]. Typically, the final traces of color disappear by 5 to 7 years of age.

Nearly normal skin is restored in at least 50% of children. The involved skin may have telangiectasias and a crepe-like laxity (anetoderma), a result of the destruction of elastic fibers. Yellow discoloration or scarred patches persist if ulceration occurred during the proliferating phase. If the tumor was once large and protruding, there is frequently a fibrofatty residuum with redundant skin. Hemangioma of the scalp or eyebrow often destroys hair follicles with resulting alopecia.

It is important to recognize that even a large and bulky subcutaneous hemangioma can regress totally, while a flat, superficial hemangioma can irreversibly alter the cutaneous texture, resulting in an atrophic patch. This variable outcome makes it difficult to predict outcome in infancy. Hemangiomas rarely cause major skeletal distortion or hypertrophy. A large facial hemangioma can, however, be associated with minor bony overgrowth, likely a result of increased blood flow. Hemangiomas can also produce a mass effect on the local facial skeleton, the nose, an ear, or the mandible.

There are two recognized subsets of hemangioma that demonstrate patterns of histologic and biologic behavior different from typical infantile hemangioma. They are both called congenital hemangiomas because they develop during prenatal life and present fully developed at birth. One type, known as *rapidly involuting congenital hemangioma*, involutes rapidly during the first few weeks or months of life [8]. These tumors are often raised with a characteristic red-violaceous color and coarse telangiectasias, often with a peripheral pale halo or central pallor. There is often superficial ulceration and, occasionally, signs of rapid arteriovenous shunting that can simulate an arteriovenous malformation. Their distribution more commonly involves the trunk and extremities. A second, less common type of congenital hemangioma termed *noninvoluting congenital hemangioma* persists into late childhood. These lesions are typically ovoid, macular, or slightly raised; pale gray in color with prominent telangiectasiae; and warm to palpation [9].

Differential diagnosis

There are two maxims to remember in the differential diagnosis of a cutaneous vascular lesion in infancy: not all hemangiomas look like strawberries, and not all strawberries are hemangiomas [7,10]. Hemangiomas are often misdiagnosed. A deep hemangioma, particularly in the cervical or axillary regions, can be mistaken for a lymphatic malformation. A macular hemangioma can have the appearance of a capillary malformation. Other infantile vascular tumors can be misdiagnosed as hemangioma, such as fibrosarcoma [11]. If there is any question about the clinical diagnosis, radiologic examination is mandated. Biopsy is essential if history, physical examination, or radiologic imaging create any suspicion of malignancy.

Clinical evaluation

Essential components of a first visit with the family of a hemangioma patient include:

1. establishment of a rapport and open dialog with the parents or care providers;
2. confirmation of the diagnosis;
3. photographic documentation;
4. consideration of the need for pharmacologic or surgical intervention;
5. determination of the need for other studies to

establish the extent of the hemangioma or to rule out associated anomalies; and
6. referral to reputable sources of information and parental support.

Parents with an affected infant, no matter how small or large the hemangioma, are understandably frightened. In general, hemangiomas arise postnatally in previously unblemished infants. Concerns include guilt over possible actions during pregnancy that may have incited this event and frustrations about how other individuals react to the child, as well as other fears of associated anomalies and of further growth of the lesion.

Reassurance is a mainstay, with open discussion of all of these issues. Parents are often afraid to raise these concerns, so a systematic review of hemangioma etiology, misinterpretation by the public, and relationship to other abnormalities is essential. It is helpful for the surgeon to openly recognize that the cause of hemangiomas remains entirely speculative and that there are no known linked factors. Parents should be told explicitly that having an affected child does not predispose them to having other affected children, but that this is a common enough entity that having another child with a hemangioma is not out of the realm of possibility.

Photographs are essential—they will provide a basis of reassurance for documented regression at subsequent visits. Many parents will present with a full set of photos documenting their emotional trial. It may be helpful to sit down and review photographic series of previous patients, documenting the course of regression or surgical results when an operation is indicated. Parents should also be referred to reputable information sources. The internet, an unedited modality, is replete with alarming Web sites, so it is helpful to guide families to respectable authorities. One particularly helpful Web site is the hemangioma newsline (www.hnnewsline.org), which is maintained by the National Organization for Vascular Anomalies. Depending on the level of concern, it may also be helpful to refer new parents to parents of previous patients who have indicated a willingness to speak with others.

The physical examination is generally detailed. Key questions to consider are:

- Is there dermatomal involvement, jeopardy to vision, a bearded involvement, or stridor in the head and neck?
- Is there ulceration?
- Are there multiple cutaneous lesions?
- Is there a lumbosacral or perineal involvement?

Dermatomal head and neck involvement. If there is a dermatomal distribution in V1/V2/V3, consideration must be made of PHACES syndrome (Posterior fossa malformations, Hemangiomas, Arterial anomalies, Coarctation of the aorta and cardiac defects, and Eye abnormalitieS) [12–14]. These hemangiomas tend to be macular with superficial skin involvement and a seeming paucity of subcutaneous tissue. In these cases, it is important to look for associated sternal notching or a midline raphe. If this is suspected, a full radiologic workup is mandated, including head and neck MRI/magnetic resonance angiography to visualize the carotids and circle of Willis, along with ophthalmologic evaluation. Reported ocular associations include micropthalmia, increased retinal vascularity, congenital cataract, and optic nerve hypoplasia. There may be persistent embryonic intra- and extracranial arteries, hypoplasia or absence of the ipsilateral carotid or vertebral vessels, aneurysmal dilatation of the carotid artery [12], coarctation and right-sided aortic arch, or dilatation of the carotid siphon.

Visual interference. In the neonate, assessment of any hemangioma that has the potential to increase pressure on the visual globe should include evaluation by a pediatric opthalmologist. Periorbital hemangioma can block the visual axis, causing deprivation amblyopia, or extend into the retrobulbar space, leading to ocular proptosis. More often, a small hemangioma involving the upper eyelid or supraorbital area can distort the growing cornea, producing astigmatic amblyopia. The results of the ophthalmic evaluation will help guide therapy.

Airway involvement/stridor. Subglottic hemangioma is a common life-threatening lesion. The symptoms are typically hoarseness and, later, biphasic stridor, generally manifesting between 4 and 12 weeks of age. Approximately 50% of these infants have a cutaneous cervical hemangioma, often in the "beard distribution" [15]. Evaluation of an infant with a cervicofacial hemangioma should include assessment of the airway. If pharmacologic therapy fails, a tracheostomy may be necessary.

Ulceration. Spontaneous epithelial breakdown, crusting, ulceration, and necrosis occur in 5% of cutaneous hemangiomas. Ulceration can arise at any anatomic site, but is most frequent in lesions involving the lips, perineum, anogenital area, and extremities (Fig. 2). The infant becomes tremendously irritable from the pain, often feeding and sleeping poorly. Ulceration may destroy an infant's eyelid, lip, or nose. Ulcerated sites may become secondarily infected, leading to cellulitis, septicemia, and, in some cases, death [16].

Cleansing, along with a daily application of hydrated petrolatum, such as Aquaphor or a topical antibiotic, is useful for small or superficial ulcerations. Topical viscous lidocaine may be applied intermittently to relieve pain. DuoDERM, Tegaderm, or Mepilex may be applied. Dressings are often

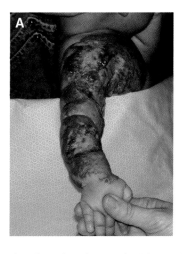 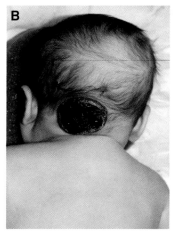

Fig. 2. Hemangioma ulceration. Ulceration may be (*A*) extensive or (*B*) localized. Surgical resection of localized, ulcerated lesions should be considered.

difficult to secure in anatomic locations where ulcerations are common.

Superficial ulceration usually heals within days to weeks, although deep ulceration can take weeks to reepithelialize. Pharmacologic treatment with corticosteroid can accelerate healing and minimize recurrence. Flashlamp pulsed-dye laser may also alleviate pain and promote healing. If possible, total resection of an ulcerated hemangioma should be contemplated if primary closure is possible and if the resulting scar would be predictably the same following surgical removal of the regressed hemangioma later in childhood. Resection in infancy is most often indicated for ulcerated tumors of the scalp, trunk, or extremity, and rarely for facial lesions. Following involution of hemangioma, scarring is predictably worse in areas of ulceration compared with previously non-ulcerated areas.

Multiple cutaneous lesions

Multiple hemangiomas in a single patient have been called "disseminated hemangiomatosis." In these infants, the cutaneous lesions are usually tiny (<5 mm in diameter), firm, and dome-like. Any infant with five or more cutaneous tumors should be suspected to harbor visceral hemangiomas (most commonly in the liver, followed by the brain, gastrointestinal tract, and lung) and screened by way of ultrasonography or MRI as indicated.

Lumbosacral disease

Lumbosacral hemangiomas are recognized to be associated with an underlying tethered spinal cord. Ultrasonography is useful for screening infants less than 4 months of age for occult spinal dysraphism. MRI is generally needed to identify spinal cord abnormalities. There are rare instances in which pelvic or perineal hemangiomas may be associated with urogenital and anorectal anomalies, such as anterior or vestibular anus, hemiclitoris, atrophic or absent labia minora, and hypospadius [17].

Treatment

Observation. Most hemangiomas are small, banal tumors, which should simply be allowed to undergo proliferation and involution. These will leave normal or slightly blemished skin. Usually, however, an infant with hemangioma is referred to a plastic surgeon because of the hemangioma's large size, rapid growth, dangerous location, ulceration, or potential for other complications.

Pharmacologic therapy for complications. The precise frequency of endangering and life-threatening complications, such as tissue destruction, distortion and obstruction, caused by hemangiomas has been estimated to be 10% [18]. The first line of medical treatment is corticosteroid, either topical, intralesional, or systemic. If the lesion does not respond to corticosteroid, second-line pharmacologic agents include vincristine or interferon alfa-2b.

1. *Topical or intralesional corticosteroid.* Intralesional injection of corticosteroid should be considered for a small, well-localized cutaneous hemangioma located on the nasal tip, cheek, lip, or eyelid to slow the growth of the tumor and minimize distortion of surrounding structures. Triamcinolone (25 mg/mL), at a dosage of 3 to 5 mg/kg, is injected slowly at a low pressure with a 3-mL syringe and fine gauge needle. If possible, the periphery of the lesion should be compressed (using the ring of an instrument) to concentrate the colloidal particles within the lesion. Subcutaneous atrophy can result, but this is usually temporary. Typically, 3 to 5 injections are needed at 6- to 8-week intervals with a response rate similar to that for systemic corticosteroid. Intralesional injection for periorbital hemangioma should be used cautiously. Blindness and eyelid necrosis are reported complications. Potent topical corticosteroid resulted in improvement in one small series of patients with periocular lesions [19].

2. *Systemic corticosteroid.* The first-line treatment for problematic, endangering, or life-threatening hemangiomas is orally administered corticosteroid (Fig. 3). Prednisone or prednisolone is prescribed at a dosage of 2 to 3 mg·kg·d. The dosage is then tapered slowly, typically every 2 to 4 weeks, and the steroid is generally discontinued entirely when the child is 10 to 11 months of age. Occasionally, there is some minor rebound growth after corticosteroid is discontinued, which may mandate another 4 to 6 weeks of therapy. Rebound growth can happen if the dose is tapered too quickly or administered on alternate days. Live vaccines should be avoided during steroid treatment. The patient should also be started on an oral histamine receptor blocker (eg, omeprazole) because of corticosteroid-related gastric irritation. Side effects do occur with corticosteroid. A Cushingoid appearance is expected, such that parents should be forewarned. This subsides as the dose is tapered toward the end of therapy. There may be diminished weight and height gain, but a period of "catch up" growth has

been documented to occur following cessation of therapy [20].

3. *Second-line pharmacotherapy: vincristine, interferon alfa.* In general, the sensitivity of hemangioma to corticosteroid is as high as 90%, with stabilized growth or accelerated regression. Indications for second line therapy are: (1) failure of response to corticosteroid; (2) contraindications to prolonged systemic corticosteroid; (3) complications of corticosteroid; and, rarely, (4) parental refusal to use corticosteroid.

Previously, recombinant interferon alfa-2a or -2b was considered as the second-line drug for endangering hemangiomas [21]. However, the side effects of this agent in infants (eg, spastic diplegia) can be serious [22], leading to the adoption of vincristine as an alternative for the treatment of corticosteroid-resistant hemangiomas by several vascular anomaly centers [23]. There is no role for irradiation in the management of cutaneous hemangiomas.

Laser therapy. Pulsed-dye laser is reserved for ulcerated hemangiomas or for treatment of persistent telangiectasias following involution. Previously, some investigators advocated prompt lasering of nascent hemangioma in the belief that this would diminish growth of the tumor [24]. However, a comprehensive prospective study has now conclusively demonstrated that when infants with newly diagnosed hemangiomas were randomized to laser or control groups, there was no positive effect of laser on reducing subsequent hemangioma proliferation [25].

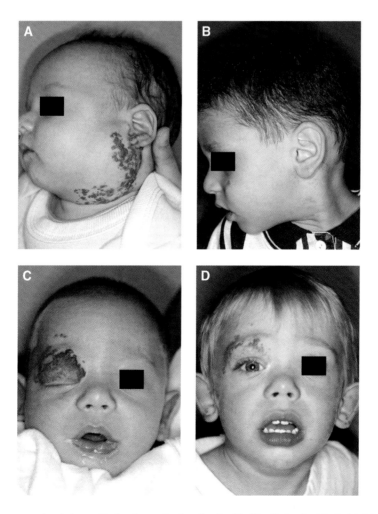

Fig. 3. Hemangioma regression in two patients who received corticosteroids. The first patient is depicted in (*A*) and (*B*), the second patient in (*C*) and (*D*).

Operative management. Excision can be considered during each of the three stages of the hemangioma life cycle for select circumstances.

1. *Infancy (proliferative phase).* Relative indications for excision of hemangioma during the proliferative phase include: (1) obstruction, usually visual or subglottic; (2) deformation, such as periorbital distortion with secondary astigmatic amblyopia; (3) bleeding or ulceration unresponsive to medical or laser therapy; and (4) anticipated scar from ulceration that would be more pronounced than that following surgical resection. Obstructive hemangiomas of the upper eyelid or brow that do not respond to pharmacologic therapy can be excised or debulked. Other respectable lesions include those that are well-localized or pedunculated, particularly those that bleed or are ulcerated. Ulcerated scalp hemangiomas generally lead to alopecia. The scalp is lax in an infant, facilitating excision and primary closure.

2. *Early childhood (involuting phase).* Typically, excision of a large or protruberant involuting phase hemangioma is done during the pre-school period. Children generally become aware of physical differences at approximately three years of age. Excision of a hemangioma in early childhood is indicated if (1) it is obvious that resection is inevitable; (2) the scar would be the same were excision postponed until the involuted phase, or (3) the scar can be easily hidden. Unique consideration must be given to every child's hemangioma. Conventional resection techniques are not always applicable. Although lenticular excision and linear closure is a traditional method for the removal of a spheroidal lesion, a circular excision with intradermal purse-string closure may yield preferable results for resection of residual protruberant fibrofatty tissue following hemangioma involution [26].

3. *Late childhood (involuted phase).* When possible, resection of affected tissue should be postponed to this phase. The involuted skin can look quite normal, particularly if the hemangioma involved only the superficial dermis. Often, though, the skin is atrophic with tiny telangiectatic vessels. Previously ulcerated areas may manifest as a hypopigmented or yellowish-tan scar. Indications for resection during late childhood include (1) damaged skin, (2) abnormal contour, and (3) distortion. Resection may be possible in a single stage, but staged

excision may be required, particularly for involuted lesions of the lips, cheek, glabela, and scalp.

Pyogenic granuloma

Pyogenic granuloma is an extremely common acquired vascular tumor in the pediatric population. These lesions can occur anywhere but usually arise in the face. Pyogenic granulomas can grow rapidly, evolving from sessile papules into pedunculated tumors connected to the underlying dermis by a narrow stalk. They generally remain small (average diameter: 6.5 mm). Frightened parents will frequently bring their child to a physician's office following a bleeding episode. The treatment of pyogenic granulomas is either curettage, shave excision and laser phototherapy, or full-thickness excision.

Kaposiform hemangioendothelioma

Kaposiform hemangioendothelioma is a vascular tumor associated with profound thrombocytopenia, petechia, and bleeding—a constellation known as *Kasabach-Merritt syndrome*. Only recently has it been recognized that this tumor is entirely distinct from hemangioma of infancy (which is not associated with thrombocytopenia) [27]. Furthermore, the coagulopathy is more appropriately referred to as *Kasabach-Merritt phenomenon*, rather than a syndrome, because the mechanism for platelet trapping is not yet understood.

The tumor is generally present at birth, although it can also appear postnatally. The sexes are equally affected. They are unifocal and commonly involve the trunk, shoulder girdle, thigh, perineum or retroperitoneum, and, less commonly, the head and neck region. The overlying skin is a brawny deep red-purple in color, tense, edematous, and warm, with ecchymosis present over and around the tumor. Thrombocytopenia is profound (<10,000/mm^3) with decreased fibrinogen, elevated fibrin split products, and generalized petechiae. In rare cases, kaposiform hemangioendothelioma can present without thrombocytopenia or coagulopathy.

Treatment is pharmacologic. First-line therapy is systemic corticosteroid; second-line treatment is vincristine or interferon. All of these therapies are less effective in treating kaposiform hemangioendothelioma than hemangioma. The mortality rate remains high, 20% to 30%, particularly for the retroperitoneal tumor. Kaposiform hemangioendothelioma often continues to proliferate into early childhood with some regression in mid-childhood.

Even when therapy is successful in regressing the tumor, long-term follow-up often demonstrates persistent (although usually asymptomatic) tumor.

Vascular malformations

Classification

Vascular malformations result from errors of embryonic and fetal development. The classification of these anomalies is based on the clinical, radiologic, and histologic appearance of the abnormal channels, which may be either hematic or lymphatic in nature. A vascular malformation can be slow-flow (ie, capillary, lymphatic, or venous) or fast-flow (ie, arterial). If there are combinations of these elements, the malformation is called an arteriovenous malformation (AVM), lymphatico-venous malformation (LVM), or capillary-lymphatico-venous malformation (CLVM).

Capillary malformations

The pathogenesis of capillary malformations (CMs) is not understood. CMs occur anywhere on the body and can be localized or extensive. Historically, they have been referred to as *port-wine stains*—a term that is now outdated. CMs have an equal sex distribution; the birth prevalence is reported to be 0.3% [28]. The cutaneous discoloration is often, but not always, evident at birth; the stain may be disguised by the erythema of neonatal skin. Facial CMs often occur in a dermatomal distribution. Forty-five percent of facial port wine stains are restricted to one of the three trigeminal dermatomes, while 55% of facial CMs overlap sensory dermatomes, cross the midline, or occur bilaterally [29]. The mucous membranes are often involved. With age, facial CMs generally become darker and can develop nodular expansion (Fig. 4). In the lower and mid-face, there can be maxillary or mandibular overgrowth with labial hypertrophy and gingival hyperplasia. In all patients with an upper facial CM, a diagnosis of Sturge-Weber syndrome should be considered on initial presentation. Cutaneous CM in the trunk and limbs is also associated with soft tissue and skeletal overgrowth, both axially and circumferentially; these, however, rarely demonstrate the textural and color changes seen in facial CMs.

CMs are often associated with developmental defects of the central neural axis. An occipital CM, frequently with an associated hair tuft, can overlie an encephalocele or ectopic meninges. A capillary stain on the posterior chest can signify an underlying AVM of the spinal cord (Cobb syndrome). A CM over the cervical or lumbosacral spine may signal occult spinal dysraphism, lipomeningocele, tethered spinal cord, and diastematomyelia [30]. There may be subtle signs of neurogenic bladder dysfunction or lower extremity weakness, and therefore, careful neurologic examination, spinal radiographic imaging, and bladder function studies are indicated [31].

Sturge-Weber syndrome

Sturge-Weber syndrome consists of a facial CM with ipsilateral ocular and leptomeningeal vascular anomalies. The capillary stain can be ophthalmic (V1) extending into the maxillary (V2), or involve all three trigeminal dermatomes [29]. The leptomeningeal anomalies can be CM, VM, or AVM. Small foci can be silent, but extensive pial vascular lesions can cause refractory seizures, contralateral hemiplegia, and variably delayed motor and cognitive development. Anomalous choroidal vascularity can lead to retinal detachment, glaucoma, and blindness. Therefore, periodic fundoscopic examination and tonometry are essential in following children with Sturge-Weber syndrome with ophthalmic examination mandated every 6 months until age 2 and then yearly.

Current management of CM is cosmetic camouflage and laser photocoagulation, but there is still a place for excision and grafting. Timing of therapy with tunable flashlamp pulsed-dye laser is controversial. In general, significant lightening occurs in approximately 80% of patients. The outcome is better on the face (lateral moreso than medial) compared with the trunk. Multiple sessions may be required. The lesion darkens again in up to 50% of patients between 3 and 4 years following treatment.

Small fibrovascular nodules can be easily excised. Resection and resurfacing with split or full thickness skin grafts patterned to fit the esthetic facial units may be required in patients with extensive fibronodular hypertrophy. Contour resection can effectively correct macrochelia and labial ptosis [32]. Orthognathic procedures are indicated when there is occlusal canting, a result of hemimaxillary vertical overgrowth, or for mandibular prognathism.

Lymphatic malformations

The pathogenesis of lymphatic malformations (LMs) is unknown. LMs manifest in various forms, from a localized sponge-like lesion to diffuse involvement of an anatomic region or multiple organ systems (Fig. 5). Radiologically and histologically, they are characterized as microcystic, macrocystic, or

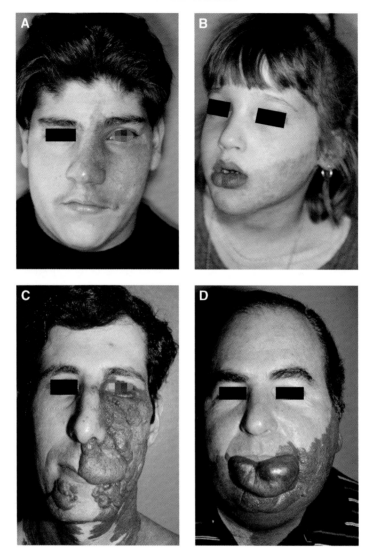

Fig. 4. Appearances of facial capillary malformation are illustrated by patients (*A–D*). Note dermatomal distribution and increasing nodularity and tissue distortion in older individuals.

combined. In the nineteenth century, microcystic LMs were called *lymphangiomas* and macrocystic LM were called *cystic hygromas*; however, these terms are outdated and should be avoided.

LMs are usually noted at birth or within 2 years of life. Prenatal ultrasonography can detect relatively large lesions as early as the second trimester, although LMs are frequently misdiagnosed as other pathologic entities [33]. LMs most commonly occur in the cervicofacial region, axilla/chest, mediastinum, retroperitoneum, buttock, and perineum. The overlying skin is usually normal, but may have a bluish hue. Dermal involvement can manifest as puckering

or tiny pathognomonic vesicles, which resemble minute blisters that become a dark-red color as a result of intravesicular bleeding.

Facial LMs are localized or diffuse, and may associated with skeletal overgrowth. Orbital LMs are reported to cause proptosis in 85%, ptosis in 73%, and restrictive eye movements in 46% of patients [34]. LM in the lower face is the most common etiology for macrochelia, macrotia, and macromala [7]. Cervicofacial LM may be unilateral or bilateral, with variable degrees of mandible involvement. LM in the floor of the mouth and tongue presents as macroglossia, vesicles, and intermittent swelling. An

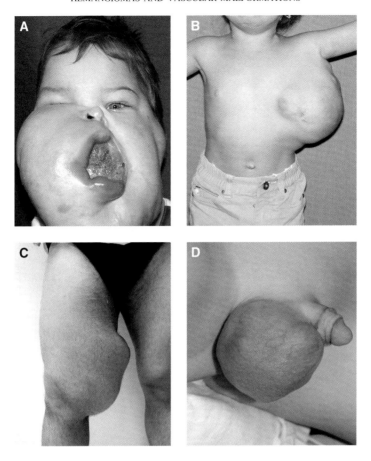

Fig. 5. Variable appearances of lymphatic malformation are noted in patients (*A–D*).

open-bite deformity generally results. In the neck, LMs most frequently occur in the anterior cervical triangle. Speech and swallowing may be impaired, and the possibility of oropharyngeal obstruction is a concern. Tracheostomy may be necessary in early infancy. The mediastinum is often involved in cervical LM.

Management of LM is directed at treating sequelae such as bleeding and recurrent infection, correcting contour, and improving function.

LMs can enlarge abruptly secondary to intralesional hemorrhage; this has been documented in 8% to 12.6% of lesions [35]. When this occurs there is sudden swelling and ecchymosis. Intralesional bleeding is a predisposing factor for infection, and antibiotics should be initiated. Cellulitis is common in LMs, particularly those in the head, neck, and perineum. This typically results in rapid expansion of the lesion with erythema, fever, and tenderness. Prompt initiation of antibiotic therapy is mandated. The clinical course may be lengthy. The involved

area often remains indurated for months. Prophylactic antibiotics are generally not indicated for patients with LMs, although parents can be given a prescription to administer the drug at the first signs of infection. Dental hygiene is an important prophylactic measure in children with facial LMs.

Sclerotherapy may be an effective therapy for macrocystic lesions. Intralesional bleomycin has a reported success rate of greater than 80% in patients with LMs of the head and neck [36]. OK-432, a lyophilised mixture of attenuated group A *Streptococcus pyogenes* of human origin, has also been reported to have dramatic results reported [37]. Its mode of action is not fully understood. It is recognized to be significantly less effective in diffuse or microcystic cervicofacial LMs [37]. Argon, neodynium:YAG, or carbon dioxide laser can be used to coagulate lymphatic vesicles on the surface of the tongue or oral mucosa [38], although these usually recur.

Surgical procedures are indicated for respiratory obstruction, nutrition, and distortion caused by LMs.

A newborn with an extensive cervicofacial LM frequently presents with respiratory obstruction secondary to involvement of the tongue and floor of mouth, which may warrant immediate tracheostomy. Resection, the mainstay of treatment for LM, can usually be deferred until later infancy or early childhood (Fig. 6). Older infants are better able to tolerate prolonged anesthesia and the dissection of delicate neurovascular structures is often easier in an older child.

Although the operative goal is complete resection, this is rarely possible because the LM involves structures that must be preserved. For a diffuse malformation, staged excision is recommended, limiting each procedure to a defined anatomic area. Reoperation on a previously resected area is teduous, because LMs frequently develop venous flow following prior surgical interventions. Postoperative wound complications are common, including prolonged drainage, swelling, seroma, and infection. An elastic compression garment should be available immediately after the procedure with refitting of more custom garments planned following the resolution of postoperative edema.

Certain surgical considerations relate to the affected region. Coronal incisions are indicated for fronto-temporal-orbital LMs. Upper eyelid LMs are removed through upper tarsal fold incisions. Hemifacial LMs are generally resected through preauricular incisions, with meticulous dissection of the facial nerve in continuity with the superficial portion of the parotid gland. Facial LMs may also be directly excised through a melolabial incision or transoral route. Labial LMs are resected through a transverse mucosal incision without violation of the vermilion border. Surgical reduction of macroglossia may be required to restore the tongue in the oral cavity or because of an open bite deformity. Skeletal contour correction with osteotomies and orthognathic procedures are usually saved for adolescence, although they can be considered earlier [39]. Cervical LMs require a radical-neck type of dissection with identification of all nerves. If the cervical LM involves the axilla, excision of these areas should be done as a separate procedure. Axillary LMs may extend into the upper extremity, necessitating staged excision; if the brachial plexus is involved, all components must be identified and preserved [40].

Lymphangioma circumscriptum is the Latin term for a superficial cutaneous-subcutaneous lymphatic anomaly, which usually manifests in the posterior cervical area, shoulder, axilla, or lower extremity as multiple vesicles that bleed repeatedly and drain clear fluid. These communicate with blind-ended lymphatic cisterns deep in the subcutaneous plane. Definitive treatment necessitates excision of both skin and subcutaneous tissue down to fascia with subsequent graft or flap closure. There is a marked tendency for recurrence.

Venous malformations

Pathogenesis

Venous malformations (VMs) are the most common type of vascular malformation. They are composed of thin-walled, dilated, sponge-like channels of variable size and mural thickness with normal endothelial lining and deficient smooth muscle. In general, they are bluish, soft, and compressible and

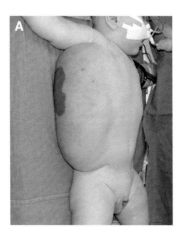 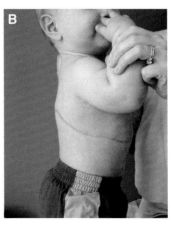

Fig. 6. Surgical resection of an extensive lymphatic malformation. (*A*) Preoperative view. (*B*) Postoperative view. (courtesy of Dr. Steven J. Fishman, Boston, MA).

tend to slowly expand with time. They principally occur in skin and subcutaneous tissues, but can also involve muscle, viscera, joint structures, and the central nervous system. They range in appearance from small varicosities to extensive lesions of the face, extremities or trunk (Fig. 7). Most VMs are solitary, though multiple cutaneous and visceral lesions also occur. The multifocal forms can be inherited.

VMs grow commensurately with the child and expand slowly, but may enlarge rapidly with thrombosis. They are easily compressed, expanding when the affected area is dependent, or following a Valsalva maneuver if the VM is in the head and neck region. Phlebothrombosis is common, leading to distention, firmness, and frequently pain in affected soft tissues. Pain and stiffness, particularly in head and neck lesions, is often most pronounced on awakening in the morning, presumably because of stasis and swelling.

Phleboliths, diagnosed as radio-opaque nodules on plain radiography, can be seen in children as young as 2 years of age.

Cervicofacial VMs are often unilateral. They can produce a mass effect resulting in facial asymmetry and progressive distortion of features. Intraorbital VMs expand the orbital cavity and may communicate with VMs of the infratemporal fossa and cheek through the sphenomaxillary fissure. As a result, the patient can have exophthalmia when the head is dependent and enophthalmia when standing upright [30]. Oral VMs tend to cause dental malignment due to a mass effect. A buccal VM can involve the tongue, palate, and oropharynx but rarely impedes speech or swallowing. Pharyngeal, tracheolaryngeal, and deep cervical-oropharyngeal VMs may compress and deviate the upper airway to cause insidious obstructive sleep apnea.

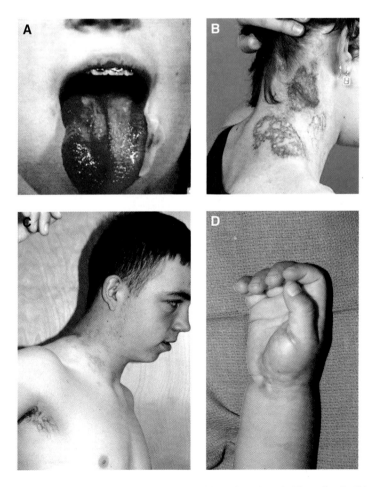

Fig. 7. Variable morphologies of venous malformation are depicted in patients (A–D). The patient in C has a supraclavicular VM that becomes evident following the Valsalva maneuver.

VM in an extremity may be limited to the skin and subcutis, or extend into underlying muscles, joints and bone, or both. Limb length discrepancy can occur, or there can be hypoplasia of the affected side due, in part, to chronic disuse secondary to pain. Intraosseous VM causes structural weaking of the bony diaphysis predisposing to pathologic fracture.

Coagulation studies should be obtained in any patient with an extensive VM, because these can be associated with coagulopathy (distinct from Kasabach-Merritt phenomenon). MRI is the most informative imaging technique for documenting the nature and extent of a VM. Venography may be required for a complete assessment in patients with extensive VM.

Indications for treatment of VM include appearance, functional problems, and pain. The principal therapeutic modalities are elastic compression, sclerotherapy, and surgical resection or a combined approach.

Elastic compression aids in reducing swelling and pain in an involved extremity. A custom garment can be worn while the patient is upright and removed during recumbency. A baby aspirin taken daily provides some prophylaxis against painful thromboses.

Sclerotherapy, the mainstay of treatment, is the injection of an agent to induce inflammation and obliteration of affected veins. For small cutaneous or mucosal lesions, local injections may be effective. For large VMs, sclerotherapy should be done under general anesthesia by an experienced interventional radiologist with real-time fluoroscopic, and often ultrasonographic, monitoring. Absolute ethanol is the most common sclerosant. Local complications of sclerotherapy include blistering, full-thickness cutaneous necrosis, and nerve injury [41]. Multiple sclerotherapeutic sessions, generally done at bimonthly intervals, are often necessary to shrink a VM because of recanalization of venous channels

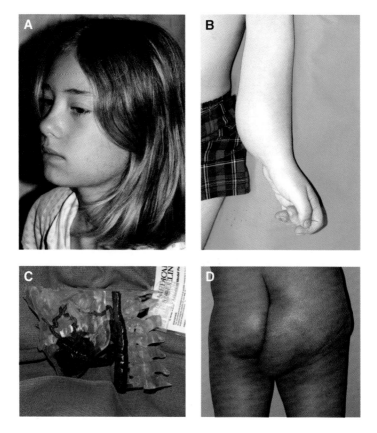

Fig. 8. Variable appearances of arteriovenous malformation are seen in patients (*A, B* and *D*). The intraosseous mandibular AVM in patient A is subtle on physical examination, but can be visualized as quite extensive in a Lucite skull model (*C*) reconstructed through medical modeling of a MRI. (courtesy of Medical Modeling, Golden, CO).

following initial obliteration. The success rate is reasonably high; in one series, 76% of patients had marked improvement or cure [41].

In general, it is preferable to shrink a VM by sclerotherapy before scheduling surgical resection. Excision of a small, well-localized VM is usually successful in these cases. In some locations, such as the hand and forearm, staged subtotal resection can be accomplished without preoperative sclerotherapy.

Arteriovenous malformations

The pathogenesis of AVMs is not understood. Intracranial AVM is the most common, followed by extracranial head and neck, extremity, truncal, and visceral sites (Fig. 8). AVMs are usually noted at birth but are frequently misdiagnosed. Usually, they are mistaken for a CM or hemangioma. Fast-flow typically becomes evident during childhood. The cutaneous stain becomes more erythematous and develops local warmth, a palpable thrill, and a bruit. A mass may expand beneath the capillary stain, occasionally with rapid enlargement following trauma or during puberty.

Later consequences of arteriovenous shunting include ischemic signs and symptoms and indolent ulceration. Intractable pain and intermittent bleeding may ensue. In the lower extremity, dry brown-violaceous plaques, known histologically as *pseudo-Kaposi sarcomas*, may appear. An extensive AVM can cause increased cardiac output and, ultimately, congestive heart failure.

A clinical staging system, introduced by Schobinger in 1990, is useful for documenting the presentation and evolution of an AVM [42]:

Stage I (quiescence): pink-bluish stain, warmth, and arteriovenous shunting by way of Doppler examination

Stage II (expansion): same as stage I, plus enlargement, pulsations, thrill, bruit, and tense/tortuous veins

Stage III: same as stage II, plus dystrophic skin changes, ulceration, (destruction) tissue necrosis, bleeding, or persistent pain

Stage IV: same as stage III, plus cardiac failure (decompensation)

Clinical diagnosis is confirmed by ultrasonography and color Doppler examination. MRI best documents the extent of the vascular malformation. AVM is characterized by the presence of feeding and draining vessels. Angiography shows variable degrees of arterial dilatation and tortuosity, arterio-venous shunting, and dilated draining veins. Feeding arteries may have aneurysms in older patients. Discrete fistulae can sometimes be visualized within diffuse AVM. In young children with diffuse AVM, a discrete nidus may not be identifiable.

The mainstays of management are embolization, sclerotherapy, surgical resection, and reconstruction. Ligation or proximal embolization of feeding vessels should never be done. Such manuevers deny access for embolization, and result in the rapid recruitment of new vessels from adjacent arteries to supply the nidus. Angiography precedes interventional or surgical therapy to precisely outline feeding and draining vessels. Embolization can be with coils or glue, either accessing the malformation from proximal arterial or retrograde venous approaches. Sclerotherapy is another approach that may be used if there are tortuous arteries or feeding vessels have been ligated. This involves direct puncture of the nidus during local arterial and venous occlusion.

Often complete resection is not possible or would result in severe disfigurement, particularly in a young patient. In these instances, embolization or sclerotherapy may be used to control symptoms, such as pain, bleeding, or congestive heart failure. Typically, embolization provides only transient improvement because of recruitment of new vessels by the nidus.

When surgical intervention is undertaken, embolization is done 24 to 72 hours before resection to provide temporary occlusion of the nidus and facilitates the surgical procedure. Extremity lesions may, in certain circumstances, be excised without preoperative embolization. The surgical goal is complete resection, unlike staged resection applicable to slow-flow vascular malformations, to minimize the chances of recurrence. The nidus, and usually involved skin, must be widely excised. Study of MRI scans, angiograms, and, occasionally, models made from MRI scans, is helpful in planning the excision. The pattern of bleeding from the wound edges is the best way to determine whether or not the resection is adequate. Intraoperative frozen sections from the resection margins may be helpful. Linear wound closure is sometimes possible. Often, primary closure requires skin grafting or tissue transfer. If there is any concern about the adequacy of resection, temporary coverage with a split-thickness skin graft can be an interim measure.

Combined embolization and surgical resection is most successful for stage I or II well-localized AVMs [43]. Follow-up evaluation is necessary for years with clinical examination supplemented by ultrasonography or MRI. The chances of recurrence are high, and experienced surgeons recognize that a "cure" can only be judged after many years. Interestingly, recurrence has been observed to involve free flap tissue used to reconstruct a defect, following incomplete excision of an AVM.

Unfortunately, many AVMs are not localized. They permeate deep craniofacial structures, infiltrate the pelvic tissues, or penetrate all tissue planes of an extremity [40]. In these cases, surgical resection is rarely indicated, and embolization for palliation is the only course.

Complex/combined malformations

Malformations not infrequently incorporate different combinations of vascular elements, such as lymphatic and venous endothelium in a lymphaticovenous malformation, and cannot be identified as purely one or the other. One example is "Klippel-Trenaunay syndrome" where patients have lesions that incorporate abnormal capillary, lymphatic and venous structures. This should, more correctly, be referred to a "capillary-lymphaticovenous malformation" or "CLVM". This malformation presents with unilateral or bilateral soft-tissue and skeletal hypertrophy of an extremity and may also be truncal. There is tremendous variability in the presentation of this disorder, from a slightly enlarged extremity with a capillary stain to a grotesquely enlarged limb with malformed digits (Fig. 9). There may be pelvic or visceral involvement. Coagulopathy is common in

patients with extensive lesions. They may be hypo- or hypercoagulable.

Treatment is aimed at the sequelae of this complex malformation, such as overgrowth, consequences of venous anomalies, and weeping from lymphatic vesicles. Overgrowth is both axial and circumferential. Limb length should be followed by an orthopedic colleague. A shoe lift may be required in early childhood with later epiphysiodesis of the femoral growth plate if there is a significant discrepancy. Grotesque congenital enlargement of the foot requires selective amputation. Massive circumferential enlargement of the calf, thigh, or buttock can be improved by staged contour resection. Hand involvement may necessitate procedures to improve function, such as digital or palmar debulking or ray resection of a massively enlarged digit. Before any surgical intervention for a CLVM, the anatomy of the deep venous system must be thoroughly evaluated. Unless a deep system is present and functioning, any intervention will predispose the patient to venous congestion in an affected extremity. An elastic compressive stocking is recommended for patients with symptomatic venous insufficiency. Treatment options for these problems include sclerotherapy, excision, and selected venous ligation.

An additional complex combined malformation is Parkes Weber syndrome, which denotes a complex high-flow AVM throughout a limb. This malformation is evident at birth with enlargement and

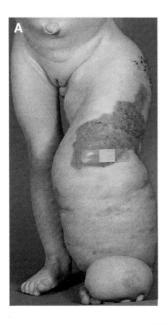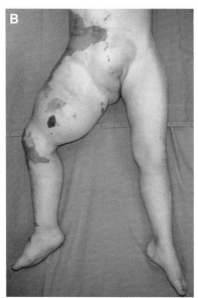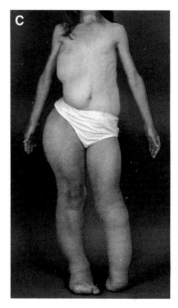

Fig. 9. Examples of CLVM, also known as *Klippel Trenaunay syndrome* are seen in patients (*A–C*).

confluent erythematous staining of the involved limb. The lower limb is more frequently involved than the upper limb. Detection of a bruit or thrill confirms the diagnosis. Overgrowth in an affected extremity is subcutaneous, muscular, and bony with diffuse microfistulae. Treatment is generally conservative, again with orthopedic involvement for the leg length discrepancy. Embolization may help with pain or cutaneous ischemic changes.

Vascular anomalies with syndromic associations

It is important for the plastic surgeon to be aware that a number of vascular anomalies fall into this category – syndromes that include both vascular malformations and other abnormalities. A full discussion is beyond the scope of this article. This includes Bannayan-Riley-Ruvalcaba syndrome, Proteus syndrome, and Maffucci's syndrome. In Bannayan-Riley-Ruvalcaba syndrome, patients have a PTEN tumor suppressor gene mutation, and develop vascular malformations and early malignancies. Proteus syndrome refers to a sporadic, progressive vascular, skeletal, and soft tissue condition that lies at the interface of vascular anomalies and overgrowth syndromes. Maffucci syndrome includes exophytic cutaneous venous malformations, bony exostoses, and enchondromas. There is a high rate of malignant transformation in these patients.

Summary

Patients with vascular anomalies were previously outcasts in the medical system. The internet has facilitated patient family communication and the advent of far-reaching support groups. With the advent of multidisciplinary clinics, physicians have found new ways to combine therapies for these complex patients. The plastic surgeon plays an essential role in defining this care.

References

[1] Mulliken JB, Glowacki J. Hemangiomas and vascular malformations in infants and children: A classification based on endothelial characteristics. Plast Reconstr Surg 1982;69:412–22.

[2] Finn MC, Glowacki J, Mulliken JB. Congenital vascular lesions: clinical application of a new classification. J Pediatr Surg 1983;18:894–900.

[3] Takahashi K, Mulliken JB, Kozakewich HP, Rogers RA, Folkman J, Ezekowitz RA. Cellular markers that distinguish the phases of hemangioma during infancy and childhood. J Clin Invest 1994;93:2357–64.

[4] Gonzalez-Crussi F, Reyes-Mugica M. Cellular hemangiomas (hemangioendotheliomaS) in infants. Light microscopic, immunohistochemical, and ultrastructural observations. Am J Surg Pathol 1991;15:769–78.

[5] Marler JJ, Mulliken JB, Upton J, et al. Increased expression patterns of matrix metalloproteinases parallel the extent and progression of vascular anomalies. Pediatrics, in press.

[6] Amir J, Metzker A, Krikler R, et al. Strawberry hemangioma in preterm infants. Pediatr Dermatol 1986;3: 331–2.

[7] Mulliken JB, Young A. Vascular birthmarks: hemangiomas and malformations. Philadelphia: WB Saunders; 1988.

[8] Boon LM, Enjolras O, Mulliken JB. Congenital hemangioma: evidence of accelerated involution. J Pediatr 1996;128:329–35.

[9] Enjolras O, Mulliken JB, Boon LM, et al. Noninvoluting hemangioma: a rare cutaneous vascular anomaly. Plast Recon Surg 2001;107:1647–54.

[10] Martinez-Perez D, Fein NA, Boon LM, et al. Not all hemangiomas look like strawberries: uncommon presentations of the most common tumor of infancy. Pediatr Dermatol 1995;12:1–6.

[11] Boon LM, Fishman SJ, Lund DP, et al. Congenital fibrosarcoma masquerading as congenital hemangioma: report of two cases. J Pediatr Surg 1995;30: 1378–81.

[12] Burrows PE, Robertson RL, Mulliken JB, et al. Cerebral vasculopathy and neurologic sequelae in infants with cervicofacial hemangioma: report of eight patients. Radiology 1998;207:601–7.

[13] Frieden IJ, Reese V, Cohen D. PHACE syndrome. The association of posterior fossa brain malformations, hemangiomas, arterial anomalies, coarctation of the aorta and cardiac defects, and eye abnormalities. Arch Dermatol 1996;132:307–11.

[14] Metry DW, Hawrot A, Altman C, et al. Association of solitary, segmental hemangiomas of the skin with visceral hemangiomatosis. Arch Dermatol 2004;140: 591–6.

[15] Orlow SJ, Isakoff MS, Blei F. Increased risk of symptomatic hemangiomas of the airway in association with cutaneous hemangiomas in a "beard" distribution. J Pediatr 1997;131:643–6.

[16] Drolet BA, Esterly NB, Frieden IJ. Hemangiomas in children. N Engl J Med 1999;341:173–81.

[17] Goldberg NS, Hebert AA, Esterly NB. Sacral hemangiomas and multiple congenital abnormalities. Arch Dermatol 1986;122:684–7.

[18] Enjolras O, Gelbert F. Superficial hemangiomas: associations and management. Pediatr Dermatol 1997; 14:173–9.

[19] Elsas FJ, Lewis AR. Topical treatment of periocular capillary hemangioma. J Pediatr Ophthalmol Strabismus 1994;31:153–6.

[20] Boon LM, MacDonald DM, Mulliken JB. Compli-

cations of systemic corticosteroid therapy for problematic hemangioma. Plast Reconstr Surg 1999;104:1616–23.

[21] Ezekowitz RAB, Mulliken JB, Folkman J. Interferon alfa-2a therapy for life-threatening hemangiomas of infancy. N Engl J Med 1992;326:1456–63 [errata: N Engl J Med 1994;330:300, N Engl J Med 1995;333:595–6].

[22] Barlow CF, Priebe CJ, Mulliken JB, et al. Spastic diplegia as a complication of interferon alfa-2a treatment of hemangiomas of infancy. J Pediatr 1998;132:527–30.

[23] Perez J, Pardo J, Gomez C. Vincristine—an effective treatment of corticoid-resistant life-threatening infantile hemangiomas. Acta Oncol 2002;41:197–9.

[24] Garden JM, Bakus AD, Paller AS. Treatment of cutaneous hemangiomas by the flashlamp-pumped pulsed dye laser: prospective analysis. J Pediatr 1992;120:555–60.

[25] Batta K, Goodyear HM, Moss C, et al. Randomised controlled study of early pulsed dye laser treatment of uncomplicated childhood haemangiomas: results of a 1-year analysis. Lancet 2002;360:521–7.

[26] Mulliken JB, Rogers GF, Marler JJ. Circular excision of hemangioma and purse-string closure: the smallest possible scar. Plast Reconstr Surg 2002;109:1544–54.

[27] Sarkar M, Mulliken JB, Kozakewich HP, et al. Thrombocytopenic coagulopathy (Kasabach-Merritt phenomenon) is associated with Kaposiform hemangioendothelioma and not with common infantile hemangioma. Plast Reconstr Surg 1997;100:1377–86.

[28] Jacobs AH, Walton RG. The incidence of birthmarks in the neonate. Pediatrics 1976;58:218–22.

[29] Enjolras O, Riché MC, Merland JJ. Facial port-wine stains and Sturge-Weber syndrome. Pediatrics 1985;76:48–51.

[30] Enjolras O, Mulliken JB. The current management of vascular birthmarks. Pediatr Dermatol 1993;10:311–3.

[31] Bauer BS, Kernahan DA, Hugo NE. Lymphangioma circumscriptum—a clinicopathological review. Ann Plast Surg 1981;7:318–26.

[32] Zide BM, Glat PM, Stile FL, et al. Vascular lip enlargement: part II. Port-wine macrocheilia—tenets of therapy based on normative values. Plast Reconstr Surg 1997;100:1674–81.

[33] Marler JJ, Fishman SJ, Upton J, et al. Prenatal diagnosis of vascular anomalies. J Pediatr Surg 2002;37:318–26.

[34] Tunc M, Sadri E, Char DH. Orbital lymphangioma: an analysis of 26 patients. Br J Ophthalmol 1999;83:76–80.

[35] Ninh T, Ninh T. Cystic hygroma in children: report of 126 cases. J Pediatr Surg 1974;9:191.

[36] Okada A, Kubota A, Fukuzawa M, et al. Injection of bleomycin as a primary therapy of cystic lymphangioma. J Pediatr Surg 1992;27:440–3.

[37] Greinwald JJ, Burke DK, Sato Y, et al. Treatment of lymphangiomas in children: an update of Picibanil (OK-432) sclerotherapy. Otolaryngol Head Neck Surg 1999;121:381–7.

[38] White JM, Chaudhry SI, Kudler JJ, et al. Nd:YAG and CO2 laser therapy of oral mucosal lesions. J Clin Laser Med Surg 1998;16:299–304.

[39] Padwa BL, Hayward PG, Ferraro NF, et al. Cervicofacial lymphatic malformation: clinical course, surgical intervention, and pathogenesis of skeletal hypertrophy. Plast Reconstr Surg 1995;95:951–60.

[40] Upton J, Coombs CJ, Mulliken JB, et al. Vascular malformations of the upper limb: a review of 270 patients. J Hand Surg [Am] 1999;24:1019–35.

[41] Berenguer B, Burrows PE, Zurakowski D, et al. Sclerotherapy of craniofacial venous malformations: complications and results. Plast Reconstr Surg 1999;104:1–11.

[42] Mulliken JB. Vascular anomalies. In: Aston SJ, Beasley RW, Thorne CHM, editors. Grabb and Smith's plastic surgery. Philadelphia: Lippincott-Raven; 1997. p. 191–204.

[43] Kohout MP, Hansen M, Pribaz JJ, et al. Arteriovenous malformations of the head and neck: natural history and management. Plast Reconstr Surg 1998;102:643–54.

Clin Plastic Surg 32 (2005) 117 – 121

Plastic surgery management in pediatric meningococcal-induced purpura fulminans

Tue A. Dinh, MD*, Jeffrey Friedman, MD, Stephen Higuera, MD

Division of Plastic Surgery, Baylor College of Medicine, Scurlock Tower, 6560 Fannin, Suite 800, Houston, TX 77030, USA

Purpura fulminans is a rare but potentially devastating complication of septic shock caused by viral, rickettsial, or bacterial infection. In children, the most common causative organism is *Neiserria meningitides*, an aerobic Gram-negative encapsulated diplococci [1]. It occurs first as a petechial rash that spreads rapidly. Once sepsis occurs, the skin rash quickly evolves into a full-thickness skin necrosis. Together with the disseminated intravascular coagulopathy (DIC), the necrosis can extend beyond the skin into the soft tissue and bone.

Children with these severe clinical presentations have had high mortality—up to 80% in several studies [2,3]. It is only in recent times, with the advances in critical care and antibiotics that allow these patients to survive, that concerns about their quality of life have become an issue. Plastic surgeons are frequently consulted regarding management of the soft tissue or the open wounds once debridement or amputation has been performed [4].

This article reviews the pathophysiology of meningococcal purpura fulminans and suggests a strategy for managing the wounds in these difficult cases.

Background

N meningitides is commonly present in the nasopharynx of asymptomatic adults. Thirteen specific serotypes exist; serotype A is most common

worldwide, whereas serotypes B and C account for most cases in the United States. The organisms become a pathogen in susceptible individuals, such as the young or the immunocompromised, by penetrating the oral or nasal mucosa [5].

The disease can manifest itself in meningitis, pericarditis, pneumonia, or arthritis. It can also occur in a mild form of acute meningococcemia characterized by malaise, myalgia, fever, and diarrhea. A rarer chronic form can last several weeks with migratory symptoms.

Fulminant meningococcemia is most severe and is associated with soft tissue necrosis. It occurs in approximately 10% of all patients with meningococcemia [6]. It presents with high fever, chills, severe myalgia, headache, and mucosal petechiae. These symptoms can progress rapidly and quickly lead to septic shock with hypotension, DIC, and severe Adult Respiratory Distress Syndrome (ARDS). The skin manifestations worsen to purpura and frank tissue necrosis (Fig. 1). This whole cascade of events has been termed Meningococcal Septic Shock (MSS) [7].

Children with MSS have the best chance for an optimal outcome in a critical care center. The care of this complex and difficult situation is best managed by a team that includes specialists in critical care medicine/ pediatrics, infectious disease, plastic surgery, orthopedic surgery, physical medicine/ rehabilitation, psychology, and nutrition service, along with dedicated nurses. Aggressive treatment has improved survival rate. Antibiotics (penicillin is still the mainstay when the organism is isolated) and inotropic and ventilatory support during the early critical period have been shown to save lives [8]. During this time, the skin and soft tissue damage is evident but may

* Corresponding author.
E-mail address: tdinh@bcm.tmc.edu (T.A. Dinh).

0094-1298/05/$ – see front matter © 2005 Elsevier Inc. All rights reserved.
doi:10.1016/j.cps.2004.09.004

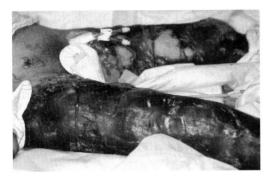

Fig. 1. Bilateral lower-extremity necrosis in a child with fulminant meningococcemia.

not be addressed, owing to the severity of the over-all condition.

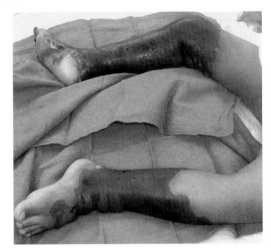

Fig. 3. Symmetric lower-extremity demarcation in a child with meningococcemia.

Pathophysiology of purpura fulminans

Hemorrhagic, purpuric skin lesions with grayish centers associated with pustules or bullae are typical with MSS (Fig. 2). In the animal model (rabbits), the Shwartzman reaction—in which localized purpuric skin necrosis occurs after exposure to antigens—can mimic the skin purpura fulminans of MSS [9]. When this is associated with massive adrenal hemorrhage, it is known as the Waterhouse-Friderichsen syndrome, which has a mortality of close to 100%. Purpura fulminans has been shown to correlate with an acquired decreased level of proteins C and S, which, together with the DIC state, leads to a hypercoagulable state in the small vessels and capillaries [10]. *N meningitides* also releases a powerful endotoxin that causes inflammatory endothelial damage, increased vessel wall permeability, microthrombi, and ultimate occlusion. The powerful inotropic agents used to maintain the blood pressure of critical patients further contribute to tissue ischemia.

The affected areas tend to be those of less perfused skin, such as the extremities. The lower extremities tend to be more severely affected (Fig. 3). The affected areas of the upper extremities are more distal and may not follow any vascular pattern. Occasionally, the soft tissues of the face or trunk are affected. The tissue losses not only affect the superficial and dermal skin layers but can also extend deeply into muscles and bones [11].

General care

Discussions should be held with the critical care specialists or team in charge. The following suggestions should be considered and instituted if agreed on by the team. They are listed in order of their relative effectiveness (with regard to tissue preservation) and of their reward-to-risk ratio as documented in the literature:

Use more cardiac inotropic and fewer vasoconstrictive agents to maintain adequate perfusion. If possible, add vasodilators to augment tissue oxygenation [12].

Maintain normovolemic or even slightly hypervolemic state if pulmonary status is stable.

Administer purified protein C. One study [13] has reported the correction of organ dysfunction in all four patients after receiving protein C, with two patients suffering no tissue loss. Given the widely accepted premise that decreased protein C level contributes to the hypercoagulable

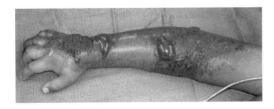

Fig. 2. Hemorrhagic, purpuric skin lesions with pustules and bullae on the right upper extremity of a child with meningococcemia.

state and microthrombi formation in the vessels, this intervention may lessen the tissue damage, although increased patient survival has not been demonstrated.

Institute blood or plasma pheresis. This procedure can improve DIC and vessel-wall integrity by removing the circulating inflammatory cytokines. Its effectiveness is anecdotal, but the risk is low [14,15].

Use hyperbaric oxygenation. Improvement of limb perfusion with this treatment has been reported [16]. The need for separation or isolation in the treatment chamber during the critical illness poses a danger.

Administer steroids. Their use has limited the hearing loss in meningitis, but it has not proved beneficial in limiting the skin loss [17]. Steroid administration in septic shock remains very controversial.

Infuse heparin. Even though heparin can decrease and mitigate the damage of vascular occlusion, the attendant risk of bleeding (already increased in septic patients) renders this treatment less acceptable [18].

Other investigational therapies, such as the administration of prostacyclin, tissue plasminogen activator, sympathetic blockage, topical nitroglycerin, or extracorporeal membrane oxygenation, have not proved very effective [19]. They also have significant potential complications.

Local care

In general, affected limbs should be elevated to decrease edema and carefully examined for compartment syndrome. This measure is especially important if the wound is circumferential or if digital examination reveals significant edema. Classically, compartmental pressure measurements of 30 mm Hg or greater have been used to indicate the need for fasciotomies. However, the mean arterial pressure must be considered; in hypotensive patients, compartment syndrome may result with intracompartmental pressures of less than 30 mm Hg. One should have a low threshold for compartment release in these patients.

The affected skin should also be examined for purulence. If purulence or abscess is present, the debridement should be performed early when the medical condition permits. During the period before debridement, the purulence should be opened to drain as much as possible, and dressing changes should be initiated. After debridement, the subsequent open wounds can be treated with wet to dry dressing changes until coverage is performed.

When there is no purulence, and the skin is ischemic but not frankly necrotic (ie, purpuric skin), the authors recommend local skin care with an antibiotic ointment.

When there is eschar or skin necrosis without purulence (ie, dry gangrene), then the skin should be treated with a bactericidal solution such as diluted Betadine (Purdue Frederick Co., Norwalk, CT) or Dakin's solution to decrease the risk of infection. The nonviable area should be allowed to demarcate before debridement. Patients with aggressive, early debridement have been shown to have a more proximal amputation level and more need for repeat surgeries than those who are allowed to wait [20,21]. The questionable areas are given a chance to recover as long as there is no active infection.

However, there is a possible benefit to early debridement of dry necrotic tissue when present in large volume: the improvement of renal function. One report exists of renal improvement after debridement of a substantial volume of nonviable tissue—an arm and a leg—in a pediatric patient [22]. This effect may be secondary to the inflammatory byproducts associated with necrotic tissue. It should be kept in mind if the patient's renal function continues to deteriorate despite optimal medical management.

The use of leeches can be helpful to salvage digits. The Hirudin effect can vasodilate blood vessels and locally decrease the hypercoagulable state, thereby increasing blood flow [23]. This treatment would be most appropriate in a patient with isolated digital ischemia.

Progressive management

After the patient has recovered from the initial critical period and the medical condition has stabilized, surgical management of ischemic tissue and open wounds can become more aggressive. The goals are still to preserve as much tissue as possible, especially the joints.

Debridements are performed to remove the nonviable skin, muscle, and bone. Even at this stage, the margins of tissue survivability can be difficult to delineate with precision. MRI, with or without concomitant angiography, can give the surgeons an approximate level of debridement or amputation [24]. During surgery, intraoperative muscle or bone biopsy can demonstrate viability of tissue. The authors' strategy is to be aggressive with debridement of skin and soft tissue (with the exception of the face), but more conservative in the resection of functional bone length and articular surfaces.

Cutaneous defects can be covered with skin grafts. However, there are reports of graft failure when grafting is performed in the early clinical course, even when the recipient beds appear ready [25]. This failure could be due to residual inflammatory response or to continued perfusion dysfunction. In the early period, when questions of tissue perfusion persist, but coverage is needed to assist in the fluid, electrolyte, and nutritional management, the authors have found that allograft skin can serve very well as a temporary physiologic dressing [22]. The allograft skin can be maintained for weeks at a time. The attachment of allograft skin can also signal the readiness of the wound to accept an autologous skin graft.

More complex defects with exposed bone or joint will require coverage with flaps. The timing of reconstruction is important. As with skin grafts, reports exist of early flap failure with both local and free tissue transfer [4,26]. Based on the literature, the authors believe that the chance of success can be increased by postponing the major surgery until recovery of local tissue perfusion and vascular integrity has occurred. This recovery may take up to 4 weeks after the initial injury. At this time, the patient should have a normal blood pressure without pressor support, and the clinical condition should be stable both in terms of infection and tissue loss. During this waiting period, careful dressing changes or temporary allograft skin coverage can keep the exposed bone and joint protected. Local and free vascularized muscle, musculocutaneous, or fascial flaps have been used with success at the authors' center and at other institutions [4,27].

Late management

Most of these patients require extensive rehabilitation and further surgical revision. One of the late sequelae of the disease is the damage to the epiphyseal growth centers of the long bones. This damage may result in asymmetric growth that will require orthopedic intervention [28]. Alternatively, the bone growth may stretch the overlying soft tissue coverage and necessitate revision. The treatment of these problems should be individualized to allow the child to lead a normal life.

Scar contracture is another frequent problem. Early treatments include pressure garments and physical therapy. Surgical scar release is frequently required and should be done early if the contracture is across a joint, so that physiotherapy can be started early. Scar release surgery can include simple procedures, such as Z-plasty to local flap rotation to free-tissue transfer [22]. The principles for surgical intervention in these patients are the same as in burn patients.

Surgical treatment for cosmesis becomes more important as the child grows. The benefits of these procedures are obvious, as demonstrated in the care of burned children. Major procedures, including the use of free flap, are indicated to allow these patients to wear a properly fitting, cosmetically acceptable prosthesis [29].

Growth and development patterns in surviving children are slow in the first 12 months after the injury. However, these patients rapidly catch up with their peers and can function well independently within their respective disabilities [21].

Summary

Purpura fulminans associated with meningococcemia is a devastating disease in children. The tissue loss can be extensive and difficult to determine at the outset. Many children survive the disease but suffer major morbidities such as amputation. The authors suggest a strategy to manage these wounds with the goal of preserving as much tissue and function as possible. At the present time, conservative therapy to the wounds appears to be the best course in the initial, critical phase, as long as no active local purulence is found. Debridement or amputation is performed when the nonviable tissue margins are delineated. Temporary coverage with allograft may be required, and definitive coverage is accomplished when the local tissue perfusion has recovered. Future revisions are often necessary and should be pursued aggressively to improve these children's quality of life.

References

[1] Rosenstein NE, Perkins BA, Stephens DS, et al. Meningococcal disease. N Engl J Med 2001;344: 1378–88.

[2] Anderson B. Mortality in meningococcal infection. Scand J Infect Dis 1978;10:277–82.

[3] Rimar JM, Fox L. Fulminant meningococcemia in children. Heart Lung 1985;14:385–91.

[4] Huang DB, Price M, Pokorny J, et al. Reconstructive surgery in children after Meningococcal Purpura Fulminans. J Pediatr Surg 1999;34:595–601.

[5] Hempel SL. Adult critical care core curriculum: fulminant meningococcemia. Overview. Virtual Hospital. Available at: http://www.vh.org/adult/provider/internalmedicine/AdultCriticalCare/FM/Overview.html. Accessed: September 20, 2004.

[6] Toews WH, Bass JW. Skin manifestations of meningococcal infection: an immediate indicator of prognosis. Am J Dis Child 1971;127:173–6.

[7] De Kleijin ED, Hazelzet JA, Kornelisse RF, et al. Pathophysiology of meningococcal sepsis in children. Eur J Pediatr 1998;157:869–80.

[8] Hempel SL. Adult critical care core curriculum: fulminant meningococcemia. Treatment. Virtual Hospital. Available at: http://www.vh.org/adult/provider/internalmedicine/AdultCriticalCare/FM/Treatment.html. Accessed: September 20, 2004.

[9] Darmstadt GL. Acute infectious purpura fulminans: pathogenesis and medical management. Pediatr Dermatol 1998;15:169–83.

[10] Powars D, Larsen R, Johnson J, et al. Epidemic meningococcemia and purpura fulminans with induced protein C deficiency. Clin Infect Dis 1993;17:254–61.

[11] Chu DZ, Blaisdell FW. Purpura Fulminans. Am J Surg 1982;143:356–62.

[12] Warner PM, Kagan RJ, Yakuboff KP, et al. Current management of purpura fulminans: a multicenter study. J Burn Care Rehabil 2003;24:119–26.

[13] Rivard GE, David M, Farrell C, et al. Treatment of purpura fulminans in meningococcemia with protein C concentrate. J Pediatr 1995;126:646–52.

[14] Westendorp RGJ, Brand A, Haanen J, et al. Leukaplasmapheresis in meningococcal septic shock. Am J Med 1992;92:577–8.

[15] Van Deuren M, Santman FW, Van Dalen R, et al. Plasma and whole blood exchange in meningococcal sepsis. Clin Infect Dis 1992;15:424–30.

[16] Dollberg S, Nachum Z, Klar A, et al. Haemophilus influenzae type B purpura fulminans treated with hyperbaric oxygen. J Infect 1992;25:197–200.

[17] McIntyre PB, Berkey CS, King SM, et al. Dexamethasone as adjunctive therapy in bacterial meningitis. A meta-analysis of randomized clinical trials since 1988. JAMA 1997;278:925–31.

[18] Kennedy NJ, Duncan AW. Acute meningococcemia: recent advances in management (with particular references to children). Anaesth Intensive Care 1996;24:197–216.

[19] Leclerc F, Leteurtre S, Cremer R, et al. Do new strategies in meningococcemia produce better outcomes? Crit Care Med 2000;28:S60–3.

[20] Huang S, Clarke JA. Severe skin loss after meningococcal septicaemia: complications in treatment. Acta Paediatr 1997;86:1263–6.

[21] Wheeler JS, Anderson B, De Chalain T. Surgical intervention in children with meningococcal purpura fulminans—a review of 117 procedures in 21 children. J Pediatr Surg 2003;38:597–603.

[22] Potokar TS, Oliver DW, Russell RR, et al. Meningococcal septicaemia and plastic surgery—a strategy for management. Br J Plast Surg 2000;53:142–8.

[23] De Chalain T, Cohen SR, Burstein FD. Successful use of leeches in the treatment of purpura fulminans. Ann Plast Surg 1995;35:300–6.

[24] Hogan M, Long F, Coley B. Preamputation MR imaging in meningococcemia and comparison to conventional arteriography. Pediatr Radiol 1998;28:426–8.

[25] Andendorff DJ, Lamont A, Davies D. Skin graft in meningococcal septicemia. Br J Plast Surg 1980;33:251–5.

[26] Misirlioglu A, Eroglu S, Gideroglu K. A rare case of meningococcemia [letter]. Plast Reconstr Surg 2002;110:993–4.

[27] Yuen JC. Free muscle flap coverage of exposed knee joints following fulminant meningococcemia. Plast Reconstr Surg 1997;99:880–4.

[28] Robinow MA, Johnson GF, Nanagas MT, et al. Skeletal lesions following meningococcemia and disseminated intravascular coagulation. A recognizable skeletal dystrophy. Am J Dis Child 1983;141:279–81.

[29] Genoff M, Hoffer M, Achauer B. Extremity amputations in meningococcemia-induced purpura fulminans. Plast Reconstr Surg 1992;89:878–81.

ELSEVIER
SAUNDERS

Clin Plastic Surg 32 (2005) 123 – 136

CLINICS IN
PLASTIC SURGERY

New developments in pediatric plastic surgery research

Randall P. Nacamuli, MD, Derrick C. Wan, MD, Kelly A. Lenton, PhD,
Michael T. Longaker, MD, MBA*

*Children's Surgical Research Program, Division of Plastic and Reconstructive Surgery, Department of Surgery,
Stanford University School of Medicine, Stanford University Medical Center, 257 Campus Drive, Stanford,
CA 94305-5148, USA*

Pediatric plastic surgery is a challenging and rewarding subspecialty for plastic and reconstructive surgeons. Although this subspecialty has traditionally been dominated by craniofacial surgery as well as pediatric hand surgery, in the last decade an expansion in the clinical treatments of vascular anomalies, nevi, burns, ear reconstruction, and pediatric urologic disorders have increased the scope of clinical pediatric plastic surgery. This review focuses on three areas of research that are emerging as important underpinnings of continued clinical advances in pediatric plastic surgery: cranial suture biology, distraction osteogenesis, and skeletal tissue engineering. We have chosen to concentrate on these three topics because they are scientific disciplines that are also of interest to pediatric plastic surgery investigators.

Studies exploring cranial suture biology are important because of the translational implications for craniosynostosis and their surgical therapies. Lessons gained by understanding the detailed biology underlying suture fusion versus suture patency may lead to biologically based therapies that can be added to our current surgical armamentarium. The current scientific models for cranial suture biology are dominated by mice and rats. This largely relates to the fact that one of the sutures, the posterior frontal, fuses early in postnatal life. We will describe recent advances in cranial suture biology in this review.

A second area that we will concentrate on is the biology underlying distraction osteogenesis. Although distraction osteogenesis began over 50 years ago in the appendicular skeleton through the pioneering work of Ilizarov, it has rapidly expanded into the craniofacial skeleton in the last decade. The initial work by Joe McCarthy and his group at NYU on the mandible has made a "march from south to north" when viewed on the craniofacial skeleton. There are numerous new devices and techniques that are undergoing clinical investigation at the time of this review. We will present an overview of the biology underlying distraction osteogenesis and predominately focus on work conducted in small animal models such as mice and rats.

Finally, skeletal tissue engineering is an exciting new area for regenerative medicine. Craniofacial surgeons and pediatric plastic surgeons struggle with insufficient amounts of bone on an almost daily basis. Current techniques for bone replacement include autografts from the skull and ribs, allografts, and bone substitutes; however, each of these techniques has associated drawbacks. Although there is no question that calvarial, hip, and rib autografts remain the gold standard in craniofacial surgery for bone replacement, they are associated with morbidities during the harvesting procedures as well as donor site limitations. The appealing concept of taking multipotent cells and combining them with osteogenic bioengineered scaffolds has a tremendous appeal for craniofacial surgeons. Recent work from our laboratory as well as others have shown that multipotent cells can indeed regenerate critical size defects in the skull. In this article we provide an overview of new

---

* Corresponding author.
E-mail address: longaker@stanford.edu
(M.T. Longaker).

0094-1298/05/$ – see front matter © 2005 Elsevier Inc. All rights reserved.
doi:10.1016/j.cps.2004.10.003

plasticsurgery.theclinics.com

developments in cell-based tissue engineering for bone, emphasizing a relatively new cell source for tissue engineering.

Cranial suture biology

Development

Normal calvarial development is dependent upon coordinated growth between the brain and overlying cranial bone plates, with fibrous joints or sutures interposed between adjacent bones facilitating much of the expansion of the skull. Minor perturbations in the complex communications between the brain, dura mater, suture mesenchyme, and osteogenic fronts during development may manifest in premature, pathologic fusion of cranial sutures. Knowledge and comprehension of these tissue interactions may eventually facilitate biologically based treatments for craniosynostosis. To better understand the molecular mechanisms governing suture biology, researchers have primarily used rat and mouse models. Both the mouse and rat systems serve well as investigational platforms with which to study suture fusion, because the posterior frontal suture undergoes physiologic fusion in a predictable manner and can be viewed as a model of pathologic suture fusion [1]. This model enables us to examine the cellular and molecular events occurring at critical time points before and during suture fusion, data not readily available from clinical specimens. Furthermore, a high degree of homology exists between the molecular genetics of mouse and man, including conservation of developmental processes and signaling pathways [2]. Mouse and rat models have enabled both in vitro and in vivo experiments to elucidate the mechanisms behind cranial suture patterning, development, and ultimate fusion or patency.

Using the power of transgenic mice, new insight into the embryologic origins of cranial sutures has recently been offered by Jiang and colleagues [3]. Previously, the embryologic origins of the bones and sutures forming the cranial vault have been unclear, with these structures presumed to be derived from the cranial neural crest (CNC) [4,5]. Using a transgenic mouse where the neural-crest specific promoter *Wnt1* was used to drive expression of *lacz* (thus permanently labeling all cells of CNC origin), Jiang and colleagues were able to demonstrate in detail the embryologic source of the frontal and parietal bones and their associated sutures [3]. The authors found that while the dura mater and frontal bones are of CNC origin as previously reported, the parietal

bones are derived from mesoderm. Interestingly, different combinations of neural crest– and mesodermal-derived tissues were found to comprise the cranial sutures, with the patent coronal and sagittal sutures forming at the interfaces between mesodermal and CNC-derived tissues. In contrast, the fusing posterior frontal suture was found to be formed entirely of neural crest cells, with both the osteogenic fronts of the flanking frontal bones, and the intervening suture mesenchyme, of CNC origin. Thus, it is possible that normal suture patterning and fate determination (ie, patency vs. fusion) are dependent on interactions between neural crest and mesodermal tissues. The data presented by Jiang and colleagues have therefore opened up another exciting avenue of research into cranial suture patency and fusion.

Genetics

Identification of the genetic basis of craniosynostosis has led to the emergence of molecular diagnoses. Diagnoses that incorporate genetic criteria as a component offer advantages including early prenatal detection, improved genetic counseling, and more informed patient management [6]. For example, a number of studies have demonstrated that molecular diagnosis is superior to clinical diagnosis as a predictor of surgical outcome [7,8]. Further elucidation of the molecular pathways involved in cranial suture fusion will facilitate the design of less invasive therapeutic strategies that will hopefully complement or replace the complex surgical procedures currently used to treat craniosynostosis.

The significance of FGF signaling and premature suture fusion has long been established, because multiple gain-of-function mutations in FGF receptors have been linked to craniosynostosis syndromes [9]. Our laboratory has previously demonstrated that higher levels of *fgf2* mRNA and protein are associated with the dura mater associated with the fusing posterior frontal suture as compared with the patent sagittal suture [10,11]. Studies by Greenwald and colleauges [12] demonstrated that increased expression of *fgf2* in rat coronal sutures led to pathologic fusion, whereas blocking FGF signal transduction in the posterior frontal suture led to a widely patent posterior frontal suture.

Iseki and colleagues [13,14] have demonstrated FGF2 to stimulate production of osteopontin and osteonectin (markers of osteoblast differentiation) in embryonic sutures, while concomitantly reducing rates of proliferation. Expression of *fgfr1*, determined by in situ hybridization, was found to be up-regulated in areas of highest FGF2 concentration.

In regions of lower FGF2 activity, both *fgfr2* expression and cellular proliferation rates were significantly increased. Consistent with the findings of Iseki and colleagues, we have recently demonstrated that both the transcription and translation of *fgfr1* and *fgfr2* are altered in rat calvarial osteoblasts undergoing differentiation, tipping the balance toward greater levels of fgfr1 [15]. These data suggest that perturbations in the relative levels of FGFR1 and FGFR2 may alter the balance of proliferation and differentiation in osteoblasts, and that such alteration may lead to pathologic premature fusion of calvarial sutures. The investigation of downstream gene activation in response to FGF signal transduction through specific FGF receptor isoforms will undoubtedly prove to be central to our comprehension of the molecular mechanisms underlying craniosynostosis. Future studies may center on FGF receptor knockout mice or mRNA silencing (siRNA) of FGF receptors to help elucidate the complex interactions governing suture fusion.

Recent studies have linked Msx2 with FGF signaling. FGF ligands delivered to mouse calvaria using heparin beads resulted in increased *msx2*, *runx2*, *bsp*, and *osteocalcin* gene expression, decreased cell proliferation, and suture fusion [16]. The coronal suture, which is the most commonly affected suture in syndromic craniosynostosis, exhibited the greatest increase in *msx2* expression and was the most likely to undergo obliteration and fusion [16]. These results suggest that Msx2 is a downstream target of FGF receptor signaling.

The association of the *Msx2* gain-of-function mutation with premature suture fusion (Boston-type craniosynostosis), and *Msx2* haploinsufficiency with calvarial ossification defects, indicates a critical role for *Msx2* in cranial development that is dosage-dependent [17–19]. Temporal and spatial patterns of *msx2* expression in the mouse are consistent with a role in suture morphogenesis. In the embryo *msx2* is expressed in membranous bones of the calvaria, cranial suture mesenchyme, dura mater and underlying neural tissue [18,19]. In neonatal mice *msx2* is expressed at the osteogenic fronts of calvarial sutures [19]. Postnatal expression of *msx2* is diminished in the mesenchyme and absent from the dura mater [20].

Studies in transgenic mice have demonstrated a role for *msx2* in the regulation of cell proliferation and support the notion that *msx2* dosage is critical for normal craniofacial development. Mice carrying an *msx2* transgene encoding the murine equivalent of the human P148H mutation exhibit increased proliferation in osteogenic fronts of calvarial bone and premature fusion of the sagittal suture [21]. Conversely,

msx2 mutant mice exhibit persistently unossified areas of calvaria referred to as calvarial foramina [22]. The defect is more exaggerated in *msx2* homozygous null mice compared with heterozygotes [21,22]. Defects in differentiation and proliferation of the neural-crest derived population of skeletogenic mesenchymal cells that compose the frontal bone have been identified as the cause of calvarial foramina in Msx2 mutants [17].

Twist is a basic helix–loop–helix transcription factor involved in cranial neural tube morphogenesis [23]. Heterozygous *Twist* mutations and deletions have been identified in Saethre-Chotzen syndrome, an autosomal dominant craniosynostotic syndrome involving one or both coronal sutures with high penetrance and variable expressivity [24,25]. In contrast to the *MSX2* and *FGFR* gain-of-function mutations associated with craniosynostosis, the frequency of *Twist* deletions and nonsense mutations identified in patients with Saethre-Chotzen syndrome suggests that the genetic mechanism in this syndrome is haploinsufficiency [26]. Mice heterozygous for *twist* exhibit phenotypic defects that parallel those found in Saethre-Chotzen syndrome, with the majority of *twist* heterozygous mice affected by complete or partial synostosis of the coronal sutures [27]. The phenotype of twist heterozygous mice indicates that the role of the twist gene is conserved between mice and humans.

Studies in mice examining the relationship between *twist* and *fgfr* gene expression have produced evidence linking them in the same signaling network during osteoblast differentiation [28,29]. The spatial and temporal patterns of expression of these genes in the coronal suture of mice suggest that *twist* may function in the suture mesenchyme to separate and maintain in a proliferative state frontal and parietal populations of osteoprogenitor cells [29]. Based on these results, it has been speculated that a decrease in *twist* dosage would reduce its inhibitory effect on osteoblast differentiation, leading to premature bony fusion of the suture [30].

BMP antagonists

Although much work has already been done to examine fibroblast growth factors and their receptors, the BMP antagonist Noggin has recently become closely associated with FGF2 activity. Already known to be involved in vertebrate dorsal-ventral patterning, Noggin has been shown to play a role in the maintenance of suture patency [31,32]. Our laboratory has recently demonstrated via in situ hybridization studies that markers of osteoblast differentiation have similar temporal-spatial expression profiles in mouse posterior frontal and sagittal sutures [33]. Similarly, comparing gene expression in fusing and patent sutures using quantitative, real-time reverse-transcriptase polymerase chain reaction, *bmp4* expression was found unexpectedly to be equivalent in the mesenchyme and osteogenic fronts of both posterior frontal and sagittal sutures [32]. In situ hybridization was subsequently used to identify possible antagonists, with Noggin expression noted to be elevated in patent sutures. Interestingly, BMP4 was found to stimulate osteoblast expression of Noggin in a dose-dependent manner, and treatment of cultured osteoblasts with FGF2 inhibited this BMP4-mediated increase in Noggin expression. Injection of *fgf2* expressing adenoviral constructs into coronal suture dura mater of immature mice demonstrated suppression of *noggin* and abnormal suture fusion. In contrast, ectopic expression of *noggin* in posterior frontal sutures led to abnormal suture patency. Our laboratory has also recently demonstrated that *bmp3*, an atypical member of the BMP family that is actually a functional antagonist of BMP-mediated signaling, is differentially regulated in fusing and nonfusing rat cranial sutures (with higher levels present in the patent suture) and that its expression is down-regulated by FGF signaling [34,35].

These data suggest that BMP antagonists such as Noggin may play a pivotal role in the regulation of cranial suture patency, possibly by acting as downstream mediators of FGF signaling. Further analysis of Noggin may be assisted through the investigation of conditional Noggin knockout mice or by employing new technologies such as RNA silencing.

Apoptosis

The balance between proliferation, differentiation, and cell death remains an active area of craniosynostosis research. Recent work has suggested a role for apoptosis in bone formation, resorption, and normal sutural development; however, the precise function of apoptosis continues to be quite controversial. Assays for programmed cell death have demonstrated both increased and decreased rates of apoptosis in vitro in osteoblasts derived from patients with syndromic craniosynostosis [36,37]. Several investigators have suggested that there is an increase in programmed cell death in sutures that are physiologically patent, while other studies suggest the opposite [36,38–40]. Recently, Zhang and colleagues [41] have demonstrated that up-regulation of the craniosynostosis-associated gene *Nell-1* leads to enhanced apoptotic rates in rat osteoblasts in vitro. Over expression of

Nell-1 in transgenic mice resulted in multiple craniofacial abnormalities, with TUNEL assays demonstrating significantly more programmed cell death along the osteogenic fronts of prematurely fused sutures. Current work from our laboratory using quantitative techniques in vivo has identified similar levels of apoptosis in both the posterior frontal and sagittal sutures during the time of predicted posterior frontal suture fusion in rats [42]. Subsequent microarray analysis of the sutures suggested that unique patterns of apoptotic gene expression exist in each suture complex, with fusing posterior frontal sutures increasing transcription of genes implicated in mitochondrial apoptosis and sagittal sutures activating genes involved in death receptor-mediated apoptosis. These data suggest that programmed cell death may be occurring by distinct mechanisms specific to each suture complex studied, and may be reflective of the different cytokine milieus and/or mechanical environments of fusing and nonfusing sutures. Despite these findings, the role of apoptosis has yet to be fully defined. Future analysis by inhibition of apoptosis or the study of transgenic FGFR gain-of-function mice may help to better elucidate the interplay between programmed cell death and premature suture fusion.

Distraction osteogenesis

Skeletal hypoplasias can effect numerous craniofacial structures, including the midface, maxilla, mandible, and neurocranium. Children afflicted with these insufficiencies of normal craniofacial development suffer from multiple disabilities ranging from malocclusion and dysfunctional bite to severe airway compromise. The necessary reconstruction of these deficiencies presents a challenge to both adult and pediatric craniofacial surgeons, because traditional reconstructive approaches present significant short-term and long-term morbidities and thus are not ideal solutions. However, the adoption of the technique of distraction osteogenesis to the craniofacial skeleton has revolutionized the treatment of many of these hypoplasias [43].

Distraction osteogenesis is a form of endogenous tissue engineering that uses controlled mechanical distraction to guide regeneration of bone in a relatively short period and yields a regenerate that is similar in size and shape to the native bone. Ilizarov first identified the physiologic and mechanical factors governing successful bony regenerate formation using a long bone fracture model in the 1950s [44,45]. This technique was first applied to the human craniofacial skeleton in 1989 as a procedure to lengthen the mandible [43]. Since then, distraction osteogenesis has rapidly spread throughout the entire field of craniofacial reconstruction, and is currently the treatment of choice for numerous mandibular and midface deficiencies [46–48].

Molecular biology

Multiple animal models have been used to dissect the general histological, structural, and mechanical changes that occur during distraction osteogenesis and lead to new bone formation. Although large animal models, such as canine, ovine, and lagomorph, have provided useful information regarding a number of these processes, these models are inherently more expensive to use than smaller, murine models and are further hampered by a lack of sophisticated molecular reagents [49–51]. Thus, investigators attempting to unravel the molecular biology regulating de novo bone formation during distraction osteogenesis have turned to murine models. Numerous studies in rats have suggested that a number of factors, such as BMP and transforming growth factor β, are involved in bone formation in the distraction gap [52,53]. Recently, Ashinoff and colleagues [54] demonstrated that bone formation during distraction osteogenesis in rats could be enhanced by adenoviral delivery of BMP-2 to the regenerate, suggesting that correct manipulation of the molecular biology induced by distraction may lead to clinically applicable therapies. A link between the mechanical environment and subsequent gene expression has recently been proposed by Tong and colleagues [55] using a rat model of distraction osteogenesis. The authors demonstrate localization of focal adhesion kinase protein, a regulator of integrin-mediated signal transduction, to areas of bone formation in distracted mandibles. No protein was seen in bone-forming, sub-critical sized defects or critical sized defects.

However, the true advantage of murine models of distraction osteogenesis lies in the development of a mouse system. As discussed previously, the genetic similarities between mouse and man make them an ideal substrate with which to work out the complicated molecular mechanisms governing mechanically induced de novo bone formation. A mouse model of distraction osteogenesis will allow what is quite possibly the most powerful tool of all to be used: that of transgenic mice. Recently, Fang and colleagues [56] have developed and validated a mouse model of unilateral distraction osteogenesis. Micro-CT and histologic analysis confirmed that successful bony bridging was achieved in all gradu-

ally distracted mice, whereas only fibrous union was seen in control mice undergoing acute lengthening procedures. The authors then used quantitative real-time reverse-transcriptase polymerase chain reaction to examine mRNA levels of several genes, including *fgf2*, *vegf*, *collagen 1*, and *osteopontin*, and demonstrated that transcripts of these genes were significantly higher in gradually distracted mandibles. This exciting work has set the stage for future investigations using transgenic mice, such as knockout mice or reporter mice, to further characterize the molecular and cellular processes occurring during mechanically induced membranous bone formation.

Mechanobiology

The mechanical environment is a key factor regulating proper bone development, adaptation, and regeneration [57,58]. This concept is one of the core premises of mechanobiology, the study of how mechanical conditions modulate the structural competence of load-bearing tissues [58,59]. Recent data suggest that a unified theory of the influence of stresses and strains on tissue differentiation is true in a variety of bone regeneration and malunion scenarios, including distraction osteogenesis [58,60,61]. This theory postulates that specific combinations of hydrostatic stress (a stress that acts equally in all directions) and principal tensile stain (a strain that represents pure elongation in a given direction) coordinates the differentiation of multipotent mesenchymal tissue into bone, cartilage, fibrous tissue, or fibrocartilage. By understanding the relationship between the mechanical environment within the distraction gap and the ensuing cascade of molecular and cellular events resulting in de novo bone formation, we can hope to modify current distraction protocols to expedite bone formation and minimize treatment times.

Loboa and colleagues [62] have recently used mechanical testing of unilaterally distracted rat mandibles to determine the stress and strain patterns associated with the lengthening phase of distraction osteogenesis, and to correlate these forces with bone formation. Their results demonstrate that strains experienced in the distraction gap ranged from 10% to 12.5% during the majority of the distraction phase, and that strain in response to distraction had a viscoelastic response, with strain peaking immediately after distraction and then gradually dropping to less than half of the maximal level. Histologic analysis demonstrated that the highest rates of bone formation occurred during active distraction, and were greatest when the nominal strains fell into the range indicated above. In a separate study, Loboa and colleagues applied sophisticated computer modeling, or finite element analysis, to distracted mandibles to quantify patterns of tensile strain and hydrostatic stress throughout the distraction gap and to determine how these patterns corresponded with bone, cartilage, or fibrous tissue formation as would be predicted using established tissue differentiation theory [63]. Data from this model revealed that mesenchymal tissue in the distraction gap experienced moderate hydrostatic stress, and would be predicted to form bone via intramembranous ossification. Tissues around the periosteal edges were calculated to be under mild compressive stress, and would be predicted to form bone via a cartilaginous intermediate. These predictions of tissue differentiation derived from the finite element analysis model correlate extremely well with histologic data from numerous models of distraction osteogenesis, including mouse and rat, where direct bone formation is seen in the distraction gap and small "tufts" of cartilage are routinely seen around the osteotomized bone, just outside of the distraction gap [56,62]. This study provides sound evidence that the success of distraction osteogenesis in engineering new bone may be mediated by the local mechanical environment created by the distraction process. Furthermore, the results of these studies are important because they provide a potential blueprint of a mechanical environment in which bone deposition is maximal. These data suggest that application of strains of this magnitude could be used in other settings requiring de novo or enhanced bone formation, such as to accelerate osteogenesis during different phases of distraction or to tissue engineer bone in vitro.

One aspect of current distraction osteogenesis protocols that may greatly benefit from strategies to enhance osteogenesis is the consolidation phase. Because the consolidation phase can represent over 50% of the total time spent in distraction, research efforts that target the consolidation phase and attempt to shorten it offer the potential of reducing device-related complications and minimizing patient discomfort [64–66]. Although the beneficial effects of mechanical stimulation of fracture callus have been demonstrated previously, few studies have investigated the consequences of mechanically stimulating the distraction regenerate during the consolidation phase [67–70]. Recently, Mofid and colleagues [71] applied a daily stimulation protocol during the consolidation phase of distraction osteogenesis that involved alternate shortening and lengthening of the regenerate. Assessment of callous volume, mineral density, mineral apposition rate, and cortical thickness all revealed that consolidation was enhanced by this exogenous mechanical stimulation. Studies such as these will prove critical to our ability to create accurate models of the effect of the mechanical environment on tissue differentiation and develop effective mechanical stimulation protocols that can be easily translated into a clinical setting.

Bone tissue engineering

Although distraction osteogenesis is an incredibly powerful tool with which to engineer new bone, the mechanical principles that lead to robust de novo osteogenesis cannot, unfortunately, be applied to every clinical situation in which skeletal repair is needed. Every year, thousands of surgical procedures are performed on the craniofacial skeleton, from the repair of injuries incurred from facial trauma to complex reconstructions due to congenital pathologies such as craniosynostosis and craniofacial skeletal hypoplasias. The national biomedical burden imparted by these procedures is substantial. In 2001 alone, over 12,000 procedures were performed on the craniofacial skeleton in children 17 years of age or younger, with an aggregate cost of nearly $270 million dollars [72]. If one includes the appendicular skeleton, the costs balloon to nearly $1 billion dollars. Thus, the need for effective strategies with which to repair the injured skeleton is apparent. However, despite our attempts to devise favorable methods with which to address these injuries, the multitude of approaches by which bony defects are treated only serves to underscore the limitations of current practice. Therapies for the repair of osseous defects run the gamut from the use of inert, alloplastic materials such as metal, glass, and polymethylmethacrylate, to allogeneic cadaveric bone and demineralized bone matrix, to autogenous sources such as split-rib or -calvarial grafts [73–82]. However, these techniques are beset by numerous drawbacks, including infection, graft-versus-host disease, failure of osseointegration, and donor-site morbidity, to name just a few [83,84]. Additional challenges are encountered in the pediatric population compared with the adult population given the constellation of comorbidities often associated with craniofacial pathology such as airway compromise.

Given the aforementioned limitations of current, traditional reconstructive approaches, researchers have sought to devise therapies for craniofacial (and general skeletal) reconstruction and repair that harness the body's innate ability to regenerate tissue. By combining the cellular and molecular lessons learned by developmental and stem cell biologists regarding the signaling processes regulating organogenesis with recent in advances in the design and fabrication of biodegradable scaffolds, researchers in the field of tissue engineering seek to create optimal clinical therapies for tissue regeneration. The quest for an ideal, tissue-engineered bony construct can be broken down into two broad categories: (1) the design and fabrication of biodegradable, biomimetic scaffolds that provide the correct molecular and environmental signals to induce osteogenesis; and (2) the identification of an ideal source of osteoprogenitor cells to seed onto the scaffold. Recent advances in these areas of research have brought the promise of tissue-engineered bone closer to the clinical horizon, making the possibility of using cell-based therapies as an adjunct to surgical treatment for skeletal deficiencies a reality in the not-too-distant future.

Scaffolds

Conceptually, an ideal scaffold for bone tissue engineering would be possessed of several properties, including osteoinductivity (able to induce bone formation), biodegradability (to allow for proper remodeling of engineered bone), biocompatibility (to eliminate foreign body reactions), and structural integrity (to provide support for local tissues). In addition, a scaffold should be easy to manipulate to facilitate design of complicated three-dimensional structures. As mentioned above, numerous materials have been described for use as scaffolds in the repair of osseous tissues, yet most of these materials are unable to meet all the proposed requirements of an ideal scaffold [85–89]. In addition, biodegradable scaffolds would, ideally, supply the necessary environmental cues to recreate a suitable niche for cellular proliferation and differentiation.

Natural scaffolds such as collagen, hyaluronic acid, and chitosan have been used as substrates for bone tissue engineering in many instances [85–89]. Recently, Cho and colleagues [89] have demonstrated that healing of canine mandibular defects treated with distraction osteogenesis is enhanced by the injection of chitosan microspheres into the regenerate, with bone mineral density increased 50% over control mandibles. However, the majority of these natural scaffolds lack the structural rigidity for independent use in areas subject to significant load, and thus may have limited application outside of treating defects with inherent or exogenous stability (as occurs in distraction osteogenesis) [90]. Much research is currently being focused on the development and testing of two types of scaffolds in particular: mineral-based scaffolds and synthetic polymer scaffolds.

Mineral-based scaffolds are designed primarily to reproduce the chemical composition of mineralized bone, or carbonatehydroxyapatite [91]. These scaffolds, which are also referred to as *calcium phosphate ceramics* or *bioceramics*, are composed of calcium phosphates, usually in the form of hydroxyapatite and/or beta-tricalcium phosphate [91,92]. Varying the ratio of these materials in the final ceramic directly affects the properties of the scaffold, most notably the rate of resorption and thus the relative biodegradability of the construct [93]. Mineral-based scaffolds have a long history of clinical use, with the first successful implementation of a calcium phosphate in 1920 [94]. In the late 1970s and early 1980s a significant push to commercialize bioceramics was made, and over the last 20 years we have seen widespread acceptance of scaffolds made from this material for general skeletal and dental use [91,95]. Bioceramics attempt to mimic the three-dimensional crystalline structure of bone and thus are osteoinductive, providing environmental information to coax progenitor cells down the osteogenic lineage, a distinct advantage over non–mineral-based scaffolds [91]. Using immunodeficient mice, both hydroxyapatite and beta-tricalcium phosphate scaffolds have been shown to induce osteogenic activity and bone formation of seeded bone-marrow derived mesenchymal cells in extra-skeletal locations in vivo [96,97]. More recently, Schliephake and colleagues [98] used preformed disks of calcium phosphate cement to repair critical sized calvarial defects in rats. Although these studies demonstrate the ability of bioceramics to induce de novo bone formation in several settings and hint at their potential therapeutic uses in vivo, widespread clinical application of bioceramics in load-bearing situations has been hampered by their structural properties. Because the bioceramics that are most suited to bone tissue–engineering applications are porous (a desirable characteristic that facilitates bony ingrowth and circulation of tissue fluids), they are inherently brittle and are prone to fracture in weight-bearing situations [99,100]. Recently, Ramay and Zhang [101], in an effort to overcome this structural limitation of bioceramic scaffolds, have developed a novel porous beta-tricalcium phosphate scaffold reinforced with nanofibers composed of hydroxyl apatite. This construct demonstrated compressive strength on an order of magnitude similar to cancellous bone. Similarly, investigators have also demonstrated increased strength of calcium phosphate cement constructs through the addition of various compounds, such as chitosan and Vicryl suture fibers, to the base scaffold [102,103]. These innovative approaches may eventually overcome the mechanical weakness of bioceramics and facilitate their adoption into clinical reconstruction of load-bearing craniofacial skeletal elements.

Synthetic scaffolds have also received much attention. The polymers most commonly used are the alpha-hydroxy acids including polyglycolic acid, polylactic acid, polydioxanone, and polycaprolactone [104]. As evidenced by the use of several of these materials as suture (Vicryl is a copolymer of polyglycolic and polylactic acid), polymer scaffolds have the ability to be extremely strong, although this strength decreases rapidly as the compound undergoes hydrolytic degradation. Rates of degradation are determined by numerous factors including local pH, crystallinity, porosity, and type of polymer; thus scaffolds can be designed with resorption times ranging from weeks to years, an advantage that can facilitate fabrication of scaffolds for highly specialized needs [105]. Although lacking the powerful inherent osteoinductive potential of mineral-based scaffolds, bioabsorbable polymers are at the very least osteoconductive and allow bone formation both in vitro and in vivo [106,107].

Currently, material scientists are combining the osteogenic properties of mineral-based scaffolds with the favorable strength and biodegradation profiles of polymer scaffolds to design novel constructs for tissue engineering. By capitalizing on advances in mineralization techniques, investigators are now able to coat nonceramic scaffolds with hydroxyapatite in as little as 3 hours [108–111]. The method by which hydroxyapatite is coated onto scaffolds can directly affect the osteoinductive capacity of the scaffold, with so-called "accelerated apatites" possessing greater ability to induce osteoblastic differentiation than standard apatites [112]. Interestingly, this accelerated apatite coating was also shown to induce expression of markers of osteoblastic differentiation in MCT3E1 osteoblast-like cells in culture media lacking typical osteoinductive reagents such as ascorbic acid and β-glycerophosphate [112]. This result underscores the importance of the composition and contour of the surface of the scaffold, which ultimately determines both the scaffold's ability to retain the extracellular-matrix secreted by osteoblastic cells and its ability to induce osteoblastic differentiation (B. Wu, personal communication) [113]. Furthermore, investigators now have the ability to combine osteoinductive coatings with recombinant growth factors onto polymer scaffolds, creating "smart" biomimetic constructs that alter their properties over time, providing temporally modulated signals to direct cellular behavior, from attachment to proliferation to differentiation. Scaffolds which combine both environmental and biologic cues for proliferation and differentiation should significantly promote and accelerate osseous regeneration.

Cellular therapies

As research into the design of optimal biomimetic scaffolds advances, we will increasingly need to determine what the biologic building block of choice will be for the design of cellular therapies for skeletal repair. Despite the interest and enormous biologic potential of human embryonic stem cells and the possibility for developing powerful new therapies employing them, this rare resource remains, for the foreseeable future, embroiled in ethical and political debates [114–116]. Similarly, burgeoning enthusiasm for devising treatments based on the delivery of genetically modified adult cells has been placed on hold because of recent complications and adverse outcomes, and continuing debate regarding the need for a possible moratorium on gene therapy [117–120]. Fortunately for tissue engineers and clinicians alike, another resource exists: the postnatal progenitor cell.

Accumulating evidence suggests that progenitor cells derived from several adult tissues including bone marrow and adipose have the capacity to differentiate into a multitude of cell types [121–123]. Whether the cells involved in tissue regeneration are "true" stem cells (which are defined as clonogenic cells that can both self-renew and differentiate), more committed multipotent or oligopotent progenitor cells, or none of the above has yet to be clearly elucidated. Such progenitors, whether delivered locally or systemically, may theoretically participate in regeneration and repair directly by giving rise to new tissue, or indirectly by either fusing with cells at the site of injury or creating an environment more conducive to the differentiation of endogenous host tissues [124,125]. Regardless of the mechanism through which tissue repair occurs, the ability to obtain progenitor cells from postnatal tissues opens up resources unfettered by the ethical and clinical drawbacks mentioned above that are associated with embryonic stem cells and the viral delivery of recombinant factors to cells from adult tissues. These properties make adult progenitor cells attractive candidates to use in cell-based therapies for craniofacial repair, regeneration, and reconstruction.

Most skeletal tissue engineering research has focused on the bone marrow–derived mesenchymal cell (BMSC) as the putative standard with which to engineer new bone [126–128]. BMSCs have been used in multiple models of osteogenesis both in vitro and in vivo, with or without scaffolds [126,129,130]. Yet despite the osteogenic potential contained in these well-characterized progenitors, several possible drawbacks may limit widespread clinical implementation of BMSC-based therapies. These include difficulty of cellular harvest and donor site morbidity, limited cell number (estimated to be as infrequent as 1 BMSC per 27,000 nucleated marrow cells), difficulty of expansion in vitro (slow growth rate and markedly decreased doubling time with cell passage), and donor-age associated alterations in biology [131–137]. Recently, however, a new cell type has emerged as an attractive alternative to BMSCs: progenitor cells isolated from the stromal fraction of adipose tissue such as processed lipoaspirate [123,138]. These cells are easily accessible, available in large numbers, and are readily expanded in cell culture [123,138]. Most importantly, these adipose-derived mesenchymal cells (AMCs) are readily differentiated down adipogenic, chondrogenic, myogenic, hematopoietic, neurogenic, and osteogenic lineages in vitro [123,138–141]. We have also demonstrated that under the right media conditions, AMCs derived from adult mice retain in vitro osteogenic potential similar to AMCs from juvenile animals, another potential advantage that these cells may have over BMSCs [142,143]. Pertinent to bone tissue engineering applications, several investigators have demonstrated that AMCs also form osteoid in vivo [144–146]. Our laboratory has recently shown, for the first time, that mouse AMCs seeded onto apatite-coated polylactic-coglycolic acid (PLGA) polymer scaffolds are capable of healing critical-sized calvarial defects in mice as assessed by histology, micro-CT, and nuclear imaging techniques [147]. No bone formation was found on any mice treated with unseeded scaffolds, or treated with seeded PLGA scaffolds lacking the apatite coating. Data from that study also suggested that constructs seeded with AMCs repaired defects as efficiently as BMSC-seeded constructs, further demonstrating the promise that adipose-derived progenitor cells hold for bone tissue engineering.

While these studies represent a critically important step forward in our attempts to design optimal therapies for skeletal regeneration, they are still potentially limited by the heterogeneity of the cells employed (be they BMSCs, AMCs, or other as yet undiscovered resources) and current biodegradable scaffold designs. However, it is quite likely that by optimizing and enriching both the population of osteoprogenitors seeded onto the scaffold and the properties of the biomimetic scaffold itself, osseous tissue regeneration can be further enhanced. More advanced biomimetic scaffolds will be capable of augmenting several stages of progenitor cell biology, including initial attachment, proliferation, migration, and terminal osteoblastic differentiation.

Complex structures

The ability to prefabricate complex composite tissue structures composed of multiple different specialized tissues may be the Holy Grail of tissue engineering. This type of technology could one day enable reconstructive surgeons to access a "spare parts" library of functional organs with which to repair or replace damaged or deficient tissues. The therapeutic potential of complex tissue constructs created ex vivo was brought into the public spotlight in 1997 when researchers at Children's Hospital in Boston successfully combined chondrocytes with a biodegradable polymer scaffold to fabricate a cartilage construct in the shape of a human ear, using the back of a mouse as a xenographic bioreactor [148]. Since then, numerous structures have been created experimentally using ex vivo and in vivo bioreactors, including cardiac and diaphragmatic muscle, vascular conduits, and urinary bladders [149–152]. More recently, Abukawa and colleagues [130] employed an in vitro rotational bioreactor to tissue engineer a mandible from a porous PLGA scaffold seeded with porcine BMSCs. Currently, one of the primary limitations of creating complex constructs in ex vivo bioreactors is the limited supply of nutrients that can be delivered to the growing tissue, because in the absence of a vascular system diffusion is the only means available. Thus, it may be that the next area of intense tissue engineering research focuses on how to induce angiogenesis and a nascent vasculature to further advance our ability to create highly complex biologic structures for the replacement of injured and deficient tissue.

Summary

Pediatric plastic surgery research is a rapidly expanding field. Unique in many ways, researchers in this field stand at the union of multiple scientific specialties, including biomedical engineering, tissue engineering, polymer science, molecular biology, developmental biology, and genetics. The goal of this scientific effort is to translate research advances into improved treatments for children with congenital and acquired defects. Although the last decade has seen a dramatic acceleration in research related to pediatric plastic surgery, the next 10 years will no doubt lead to novel treatment strategies with improved clinical outcomes.

Acknowledgments

This work was supported by NIH R01-13194 and the Oak Foundation to MTL and an ACS Scholarship to RPN.

References

[1] Moss ML. Fusion of the frontal suture in the rat. Am J Anat 1958;102:141–66.

[2] Waterston RH, Lindblad-Toh K, Birney E, et al. Initial sequencing and comparative analysis of the mouse genome. Nature 2002;420:520–62.

[3] Jiang X, Iseki S, Maxson RE, Sucov HM, Morriss-Kay GM. Tissue origins and interactions in the mammalian skull vault. Dev Biol 2002;241:106–16.

[4] Noden DM. Craniofacial development: new views on old problems. Anat Rec 1984;208:1–13.

[5] Couly GF, Coltey PM, Le Douarin NM. The triple origin of skull in higher vertebrates: a study in quail-chick chimeras. Development 1993;117:409–29.

[6] Ferreira JC, Carter SM, Bernstein PS, et al. Second-trimester molecular prenatal diagnosis of sporadic apert syndrome following suspicious ultrasound findings. Ultrasound Obstet Gynecol 1999;14:426–30.

[7] Cassileth LB, Bartlett SP, Glat PM, et al. Clinical characteristics of patients with unicoronal synostosis and mutations of fibroblast growth factor receptor 3: a preliminary report. Plast Reconstr Surg 2001;108:1849–54.

[8] von Gernet S, Golla A, Ehrenfels Y, et al. Genotype-phenotype analysis in apert syndrome suggests opposite effects of the two recurrent mutations on syndactyly and outcome of craniofacial surgery. Clin Genet 2000;57:137–9.

[9] Wilkie AO. Craniosynostosis: genes and mechanisms. Hum Mol Genet 1997;6:1647–56.

[10] Mehrara BJ, Mackool RJ, McCarthy JG, et al. Immunolocalization of basic fibroblast growth factor and fibroblast growth factor receptor-1 and receptor-2 in rat cranial sutures. Plast Reconstr Surg 1998;102:1805–17.

[11] Greenwald JA, Mehrara BJ, Spector JA, et al. Regional differentiation of cranial suture-associated dura mater in vivo and in vitro: implications for suture fusion and patency. J Bone Miner Res 2000;15:2413–30.

[12] Greenwald JA, Mehrara BJ, Spector JA, et al. In vivo modulation of fgf biological activity alters cranial suture fate. Am J Pathol 2001;158:441–52.

[13] Iseki S, Wilkie AO, Morriss-Kay GM. Fgfr1 and fgfr2 have distinct differentiation- and proliferation-related roles in the developing mouse skull vault. Development 1999;126:5611–20.

[14] Iseki S, Wilkie AO, Heath JK, et al. Fgfr2 and osteopontin domains in the developing skull vault are mutually exclusive and can be altered by locally applied fgf2. Development 1997;124:3375–84.

[15] Song HM, Nacamuli RP, Xia W, et al. High-dose retinoic acid modulates rat calvarial osteoblast biology. J Cell Phys 2005;202(1):255–62.

[16] Ignelzi Jr MA, Wang W, Young AT. Fibroblast growth factors lead to increased msx2 expression and fusion in calvarial sutures. J Bone Miner Res 2003;18:751–9.

[17] Wilkie AOM, Tang Z, Elanko N, et al. Functional haploinsufficiency of the human homeobox gene msx2 causes defects in skull ossification. Nat Genet 2000;24:387–90.

[18] Jabs EW, Muller U, Li X, et al. A mutation in the homeodomain of the human msx2 gene in a family affected with autosomal dominant craniosynostosis. Cell 1993;75:443–50.

[19] Kim HJ, Rice DP, Kettunen PJ, et al. Fgf-, bmp- and shh-mediated signalling pathways in the regulation of cranial suture morphogenesis and calvarial bone development. Development 1998;125:1241–51.

[20] Liu YH, Tang Z, Kundu RK, et al. Msx2 gene dosage influences the number of proliferative osteogenic cells in growth centers of the developing murine skull: a possible mechanism for msx2-mediated craniosynostosis in humans. Dev Biol 1999;205:260–74.

[21] Satokata I, Ma L, Ohshima H, et al. Msx2 deficiency in mice causes pleiotropic defects in bone growth and ectodermal organ formation. Nat Genet 2000;24:391–5.

[22] Ishii M, Merrill AE, Chan YS, et al. Msx2 and twist cooperatively control the development of the neural crest-derived skeletogenic mesenchyme of the murine skull vault. Development 2003;130:6131–42.

[23] Chen ZF, Behringer RR. Twist is required in head mesenchyme for cranial neural tube morphogenesis. Genes Dev 1995;9:686–99.

[24] el Ghouzzi V, Le Merrer M, Perrin-Schmitt F, et al. Mutations of the twist gene in the saethre-chotzen syndrome. Nat Genet 1997;15:42–6.

[25] Howard TD, Paznekas WA, Green ED, et al. Mutations in twist, a basic helix-loop-helix transcription factor, in saethre-chotzen syndrome. Nat Genet 1997;15:36–41.

[26] Gripp KW, Zackai EH, Stolle CA. Mutations in the human twist gene. Hum Mutat 2000;15:150–5.

[27] Carver EA, Oram KF, Gridley T. Craniosynostosis in twist heterozygous mice: a model for saethre-chotzen syndrome. Anat Rec 2002;268:90–2.

[28] Rice DP, Aberg T, Chan Y, et al. Integration of fgf and twist in calvarial bone and suture development. Development 2000;127:1845–55.

[29] Johnson D, Iseki S, Wilkie AO, et al. Expression patterns of twist and fgfr1, -2 and -3 in the developing

mouse coronal suture suggest a key role for twist in suture initiation and biogenesis. Mech Dev 2000;91: 341–5.

[30] Bialek P, Kern B, Yang X, et al. A twist code determines the onset of osteoblast differentiation. Dev Cell 2004;6:423–35.

[31] McMahon JA, Takada S, Zimmerman LB, et al. Noggin-mediated antagonism of bmp signaling is required for growth and patterning of the neural tube and somite. Genes Dev 1998;12:1438–52.

[32] Warren SM, Brunet LJ, Harland RM, et al. The bmp antagonist noggin regulates cranial suture fusion. Nature 2003;422:625–9.

[33] Nacamuli RP, Fong KD, Warren SM, et al. Markers of osteoblast differentiation in fusing and nonfusing cranial sutures. Plast Reconstr Surg 2003;112: 1328–35.

[34] Daluiski A, Engstrand T, Bahamonde ME, et al. Bone morphogenetic protein-3 is a negative regulator of bone density. Nat Genet 2001;27:84–8.

[35] Nacamuli RP, Fong KD, Lenton KA, et al. Expression and possible mechanisms of regulation of bmp3 in rat cranial sutures. Plas Recon Surg, Accepted for publication.

[36] Lemonnier J, Hay E, Delannoy P, et al. Increased osteoblast apoptosis in apert craniosynostosis: role of protein kinase c and interleukin-1. Am J Pathol 2001;158:1833–42.

[37] Dry GM, Yasinskaya YI, Williams JK, et al. Inhibition of apoptosis: a potential mechanism for syndromic craniosynostosis. Plast Reconstr Surg 2001; 107:425–32.

[38] Furtwangler JA, Hall SH, Koskinen-Moffett LK. Sutural morphogenesis in the mouse calvaria: the role of apoptosis. Acta Anat (Basel) 1985;124:74–80.

[39] Opperman LA, Adab K, Gakunga PT. Transforming growth factor-beta 2 and tgf-beta 3 regulate fetal rat cranial suture morphogenesis by regulating rates of cell proliferation and apoptosis. Dev Dyn 2000;219: 237–47.

[40] Agresti M, Schaefer RB, Recinos RF, et al. Detection of apoptosis in normal postantal mouse cranial sutures. Las Vegas (NV): Plastic Surgery Research Council; 2003.

[41] Zhang X, Carpenter D, Bokui N, et al. Overexpression of nell-1, a craniosynostosis-associated gene, induces apoptosis in osteoblasts during craniofacial development. J Bone Miner Res 2003;18:2126–34.

[42] Fong KD, Song HM, Nacamuli RP, et al. Apoptosis in a rodent model of cranial suture fusion: in situ imaging and gene expression analysis. Plast Reconstr Surg 2004;113:2037–47.

[43] McCarthy JG, Schreiber J, Karp N, et al. Lengthening the human mandible by gradual distraction. Plast Reconstr Surg 1992;89:1–8.

[44] Ilizarov GA, Ledyaev VI. The replacement of long tubular bone defects by lengthening distraction osteotomy of one of the fragments. 1969. Clin Orthop 1992;7–10.

[45] Ilizarov G. Clinical application of the tension-stress effect for limb lengthening. Clin Orthop 1990;8–26.

[46] McCarthy J. The role of distraction osteogenesis in the reconstruction of the mandible in unilateral craniofacial microsomia. Clin Plast Surg 1994;21: 625–31.

[47] Gosain AK. Distraction osteogenesis of the craniofacial skeleton. Plast Reconstr Surg 2001;107: 278–80.

[48] Cohen SR, Burstein FD, Williams JK. The role of distraction osteogenesis in the management of craniofacial disorders. Ann Acad Med Singapore 1999; 28:728–38.

[49] Aronson J. Experimental and clinical experience with distraction osteogenesis. Cleft Palate Craniofac J 1994;31:473–81.

[50] Karaharju-Suvanto T, Karaharju EO, Ranta R. Mandibular distraction. An experimental study on sheep. J Craniomaxillofac Surg 1990;18:280–3.

[51] Califano L, Cortese A, Zupi A, et al. Mandibular lengthening by external distraction: an experimental study in the rabbit. J Oral Maxillofac Surg 1994;52: 1179–83.

[52] Sato M, Ochi T, Nakase T, et al. Mechanical tension-stress induces expression of bone morphogenetic protein (bmp)-2 and bmp-4, but not bmp-6, bmp-7, and gdf-5 mrna, during distraction osteogenesis. J Bone Miner Res 1999;14:1084–95.

[53] Mehrara BJ, Rowe NM, Steinbrech DS, et al. Rat mandibular distraction osteogenesis: II. Molecular analysis of transforming growth factor beta-1 and osteocalcin gene expression. Plast Reconstr Surg 1999;103:536–47.

[54] Ashinoff RL, Cetrulo Jr CL, Galiano RD, et al. Bone morphogenic protein-2 gene therapy for mandibular distraction osteogenesis. Ann Plast Surg 2004;52: 585–90.

[55] Tong L, Buchman SR, Ignelzi Jr MA, et al. Focal adhesion kinase expression during mandibular distraction osteogenesis: evidence for mechanotransduction. Plast Reconstr Surg 2003;111:211–22.

[56] Fang TD, Nacamuli RP, Song HM, et al. Creation and characterization of a mouse model of mandibular distraction osteogenesis. Bone 2004;34:1004–12.

[57] Prendergast PJ. Finite element models in tissue mechanics and orthopaedic implant design. Clin Biomech (Bristol, Avon) 1997;12:343–66.

[58] Carter DR, Beaupre GS, Giori NJ, et al. Mechanobiology of skeletal regeneration. Clin Orthop 1998: S41–55.

[59] van der Meulen MC, Huiskes R. Why mechanobiology? A survey article. J Biomech 2002;35:401–14.

[60] Carter DR, Blenman PR, Beaupre GS. Correlations between mechanical stress history and tissue differentiation in initial fracture healing. J Orthop Res 1988;6:736–48.

[61] Loboa EG, Beaupre GS, Carter DR. Mechanobiology of initial pseudarthrosis formation with oblique fractures. J Orthop Res 2001;19:1067–72.

[62] Loboa EG, Fang TD, Warren SM, et al. Mechanobiology of mandibular distraction osteogenesis: Experimental analyses with a rat model. Bone 2004;34:336–43.

[63] Loboa E, Fang TD, Parker DW, et al. Mechanobiology of mandibular distraction osteogenesis—finite element analyses with a rat model. J Orthop Res, Accepted for publication.

[64] Ortiz Monasterio F, Molina F, Andrade L, et al. Simultaneous mandibular and maxillary distraction in hemifacial microsomia in adults: avoiding occlusal disasters. Plast Reconstr Surg 1997;100:852–61.

[65] Mofid MM, Manson PN, Robertson BC, et al. Craniofacial distraction osteogenesis: a review of 3278 cases. Plast Reconstr Surg 2001;108:1103–14.

[66] Cho BC, Park JW, Baik BS, et al. Clinical application of injectable calcium sulfate on early bony consolidation in distraction osteogenesis for the treatment of craniofacial microsomia. J Craniofac Surg 2002;13:465–75.

[67] De Bastiani G, Aldegheri R, Renzi-Brivio L, et al. Limb lengthening by callus distraction (callotasis). J Pediatr Orthop 1987;7:129–34.

[68] Lazo-Zbikowski J, Aguilar F, Mozo F, et al. Biocompression external fixation. Sliding external osteosynthesis. Clin Orthop 1986:169–84.

[69] Dehne R, Metz CW, Deffer PA, et al. Nonoperative treatment of the fractured tibia by immediate weight bearing. J Trauma 1961;1:514–35.

[70] Pandey R, White SH, Kenwright J. Callus distraction in ollier's disease. Acta Orthop Scand 1995;66:479–80.

[71] Mofid MM, Inoue N, Atabey A, et al. Callus stimulation in distraction osteogenesis. Plast Reconstr Surg 2002;109:1621–9.

[72] Steiner C, Elixhauser A, Schnaier J. The healthcare cost and utilization project: an overview. Eff Clin Pract 2002;5:143–51.

[73] Moss SD, Joganic E, Manwaring KH, et al. Transplanted demineralized bone graft in cranial reconstructive surgery. Pediatr Neurosurg 1995;23:199–204.

[74] Goodrich JT, Argamaso R, Hall CD. Split-thickness bone grafts in complex craniofacial reconstructions. Pediatr Neurosurg 1992;18:195–201.

[75] Shenaq SM. Reconstruction of complex cranial and craniofacial defects utilizing iliac crest-internal oblique microsurgical free flap. Microsurgery 1988;9:154–8.

[76] Marchac D. Split-rib grafts in craniofacial surgery. Plast Reconstr Surg 1982;69:566–7.

[77] Bruens ML, Pieterman H, de Wijn JR, et al. Porous polymethylmethacrylate as bone substitute in the craniofacial area. J Craniofac Surg 2003;14:63–8.

[78] Dean D, Topham NS, Rimnac C, et al. Osseointegration of preformed polymethylmethacrylate craniofacial prostheses coated with bone marrow-impregnated poly (dl-lactic-co-glycolic acid) foam. Plast Reconstr Surg 1999;104:705–12.

[79] Nicholson JW. Glass-ionomers in medicine and dentistry. Proc Inst Mech Eng [H] 1998;212:121–6.

[80] Rah DK. Art of replacing craniofacial bone defects. Yonsei Med J 2000;41:756–65.

[81] Hassler W, Zentner J. Radical osteoclastic craniectomy in sagittal synostosis. Neurosurgery 1990;27:539.

[82] Sirola K. Regeneration of defects in the calvaria. Ann Med Exp Biol Fenn 1960;38:1–87.

[83] Mulliken JB, Glowacki J. Induced osteogenesis for repair and construction in the craniofacial region. Plast Reconstr Surg 1980;65:553–60.

[84] Bostrom R, Mikos A. Tissue engineering of bone. In: Atala A, Mooney DJ, Vacanti JP, et al, editors. Synthetic biodegradable polymer scaffolds. Boston: Birkhauser; 1997. p. 215–34.

[85] Saadeh PB, Khosla RK, Mehrara BJ, et al. Repair of a critical size defect in the rat mandible using allogenic type i collagen. J Craniofac Surg 2001;12:573–9.

[86] Seol YJ, Lee JY, Park YJ, et al. Chitosan sponges as tissue engineering scaffolds for bone formation. Biotechnol Lett 2004;26:1037–41.

[87] Bumgardner JD, Wiser R, Gerard PD, et al. Chitosan: potential use as a bioactive coating for orthopaedic and craniofacial/dental implants. J Biomater Sci Polym Ed 2003;14:423–38.

[88] Solchaga LA, Gao J, Dennis JE, et al. Treatment of osteochondral defects with autologous bone marrow in a hyaluronan-based delivery vehicle. Tissue Eng 2002;8:333–47.

[89] Cho BC, Kim JY, Lee JH, et al. The bone regenerative effect of chitosan microsphere-encapsulated growth hormone on bony consolidation in mandibular distraction osteogenesis in a dog model. J Craniofac Surg 2004;15:299–311.

[90] Zhang Y, Zhang M. Synthesis and characterization of macroporous chitosan/calcium phosphate composite scaffolds for tissue engineering. J Biomed Mater Res 2001;55:304–12.

[91] LeGeros RZ. Properties of osteoconductive biomaterials: calcium phosphates. Clin Orthop 2002:81–98.

[92] Osborn JF, Newesely H. The material science of calcium phosphate ceramics. Biomaterials 1980;1:108–11.

[93] Blokhuis TJ, Termaat MF, den Boer FC, et al. Properties of calcium phosphate ceramics in relation to their in vivo behavior. J Trauma 2000;48:179–86.

[94] Albee FH. Studies in bone growth: triple cap as a stimulus to osteogenesis. Ann Surg 1920;71:32–6.

[95] Groot KD. Bioceramics of calcium phosphate. Boca Raton (FL): CRC Press; 1983.

[96] Ducheyne P. Bioceramics: material characteristics versus in vivo behavior. J Biomed Mater Res 1987;21:219–36.

[97] Yaszemski MJ, Payne RG, Hayes WC, et al. Evolution of bone transplantation: molecular, cellular and tissue strategies to engineer human bone. Biomaterials 1996;17:175–85.

[98] Schliephake H, Gruber R, Dard M, et al. Repair of calvarial defects in rats by prefabricated hydroxyapa-

tite cement implants. J Biomed Mater Res 2004;
69A:382–90.

[99] Boo JS, Yamada Y, Okazaki Y, et al. Tissue-engineered bone using mesenchymal stem cells and a biodegradable scaffold. J Craniofac Surg 2002;13:231–9.

[100] Harris CT, Cooper LF. Comparison of bone graft matrices for human mesenchymal stem cell-directed osteogenesis. J Biomed Mater Res 2004;68A:747–55.

[101] Ramay HR, Zhang M. Biphasic calcium phosphate nanocomposite porous scaffolds for load-bearing bone tissue engineering. Biomaterials 2004;25:5171–80.

[102] Xu HH, Simon Jr CG. Self-hardening calcium phosphate composite scaffold for bone tissue engineering. J Orthop Res 2004;22:535–43.

[103] Xu HH, Quinn JB, Takagi S, et al. Synergistic reinforcement of in situ hardening calcium phosphate composite scaffold for bone tissue engineering. Biomaterials 2004;25:1029–37.

[104] Lanza RP, Langer RS, Vacanti J. Principles of tissue engineering. 2nd edition. San Diego (CA): Academic Press; 2000.

[105] Behravesh E, Yasko AW, Engel PS, et al. Synthetic biodegradable polymers for orthopaedic applications. Clin Orthop 1999:S118–29.

[106] Ishaug SL, Crane GM, Miller MJ, et al. Bone formation by three-dimensional stromal osteoblast culture in biodegradable polymer scaffolds. J Biomed Mater Res 1997;36:17–28.

[107] Ishaug SL, Yaszemski MJ, Bizios R, et al. Osteoblast function on synthetic biodegradable polymers. J Biomed Mater Res 1994;28:1445–53.

[108] Barrere F, van der Valk CM, Dalmeijer RA, et al. Osteogenecity of octacalcium phosphate coatings applied on porous metal implants. J Biomed Mater Res 2003;66A:779–88.

[109] Barrere F, Layrolle P, Van Blitterswijk C, et al. Biomimetic coatings on titanium: a crystal growth study of octacalcium phosphate. J Mater Sci Mater Med 2001;6:529–34.

[110] Kokubo T, Kim HM, Kawashita M. Novel bioactive materials with different mechanical properties. Biomaterials 2003;24:2161–75.

[111] Chou YF, Chiou WA, Xu Y, et al. The effect of pH on the structural evolution of accelerated biomimetic apatite. Biomaterials 2004;25:5323–31.

[112] Chou YF, Huan W, Dunn JC, et al. The effect of biomimetic apatite structure on osteoblast viability, proliferation, and gene expression. Biomaterials 2005;26(3):285–95.

[113] Yang Y, Magnay J, Cooling L, et al. Effects of substrate characteristics on bone cell response to the mechanical environment. Med Biol Eng Comput 2004;42:22–9.

[114] Bahadur G. The moral status of the embryo: the human embryo in the UK Human Fertilisation and Embryology (Research Purposes) Regulation 2001 debate. Reprod Biomed Online 2003;7:12–6.

[115] Chin JJ. Ethical issues in stem cell research. Med J Malaysia 2003;58(Suppl A):111–8.

[116] Weissman IL. Stem cells—scientific, medical, and political issues. N Engl J Med 2002;346:1576–9.

[117] Dixon N. Cancer scare hits gene cures: a second major setback for medicine's most pioneering treatment has split the scientific community Could a moratorium do more harm than good? New Sci 2002;176:4–5.

[118] Grilley BJ, Gee AP. Gene transfer: regulatory issues and their impact on the clinical investigator and the good manufacturing production facility. Cytotherapy 2003;5:197–207.

[119] Smith L, Byers JF. Gene therapy in the post-gelsinger era. JONAS Healthc Law Ethics Regul 2002;4:104–10.

[120] Verma IM. A voluntary moratorium? Mol Ther 2003;7:141.

[121] Forbes SJ, Poulsom R, Wright NA. Hepatic and renal differentiation from blood-borne stem cells. Gene Ther 2002;9:625–30.

[122] Pittenger MF, Mackay AM, Beck SC, et al. Multilineage potential of adult human mesenchymal stem cells. Science 1999;284:143–7.

[123] Zuk PA, Zhu M, Ashjian P, et al. Human adipose tissue is a source of multipotent stem cells. Mol Biol Cell 2002;13:4279–95.

[124] Wagers AJ, Weissman IL. Plasticity of adult stem cells. Cell 2004;116:639–48.

[125] Wagers AJ, Sherwood RI, Christensen JL, et al. Little evidence for developmental plasticity of adult hematopoietic stem cells. Science 2002;297:2256–9.

[126] Rickard DJ, Sullivan TA, Shenker BJ, et al. Induction of rapid osteoblast differentiation in rat bone marrow stromal cell cultures by dexamethasone and bmp-2. Dev Biol 1994;161:218–28.

[127] Long MW, Robinson JA, Ashcraft EA, et al. Regulation of human bone marrow-derived osteoprogenitor cells by osteogenic growth factors. J Clin Invest 1995;95:881–7.

[128] Ohgushi H, Caplan AI. Stem cell technology and bioceramics: from cell to gene engineering. J Biomed Mater Res 1999;48:913–27.

[129] Dennis JE, Haynesworth SE, Young RG, et al. Osteogenesis in marrow-derived mesenchymal cell porous ceramic composites transplanted subcutaneously: effect of fibronectin and laminin on cell retention and rate of osteogenic expression. Cell Transplant 1992;1:23–32.

[130] Abukawa H, Terai H, Hannouche D, et al. Formation of a mandibular condyle in vitro by tissue engineering. J Oral Maxillofac Surg 2003;61:94–100.

[131] Cicuttini FM, Welch K, Boyd AW. Characterization of cd34 + hla-dr-cd38 + and cd34 + hla-dr-cd38- progenitor cells from human umbilical cord blood. Growth Factors 1994;10:127–34.

[132] Banfi A, Muraglia A, Dozin B, et al. Proliferation kinetics and differentiation potential of ex vivo expanded human bone marrow stromal cells: impli-

cations for their use in cell therapy. Exp Hematol 2000;28:707–15.

[133] Bergman RJ, Gazit D, Kahn AJ, et al. Age-related changes in osteogenic stem cells in mice. J Bone Miner Res 1996;11:568–77.

[134] Stenderup K, Justesen J, Clausen C, et al. Aging is associated with decreased maximal life span and accelerated senescence of bone marrow stromal cells. Bone 2003;33:919–26.

[135] Stenderup K, Rosada C, Justesen J, et al. Aged human bone marrow stromal cells maintaining bone forming capacity in vivo evaluated using an improved method of visualization. Biogerontology 2004;5:107–18.

[136] Mendes SC, Tibbe JM, Veenhof M, et al. Bone tissue-engineered implants using human bone marrow stromal cells: effect of culture conditions and donor age. Tissue Eng 2002;8:911–20.

[137] Mueller SM, Glowacki J. Age-related decline in the osteogenic potential of human bone marrow cells cultured in three-dimensional collagen sponges. J Cell Biochem 2001;82:583–90.

[138] Zuk PA, Zhu M, Mizuno H, et al. Multilineage cells from human adipose tissue: implications for cell-based therapies. Tissue Eng 2001;7:211–28.

[139] Cousin B, Andre M, Arnaud E, et al. Reconstitution of lethally irradiated mice by cells isolated from adipose tissue. Biochem Biophys Res Commun 2003; 301:1016–22.

[140] Huang JI, Beanes SR, Zhu M, et al. Rat extramedullary adipose tissue as a source of osteochondrogenic progenitor cells. Plast Reconstr Surg 2002;109: 1033–41.

[141] Gimble JM, Guilak F. Differentiation potential of adipose derived adult stem (adas) cells. Curr Top Dev Biol 2003;58:137–60.

[142] Shi Y, Nacamuli RP, Salim A, et al. The osteogenic potential of adipose-derived mesenchymal cells is maintained with aging. Plast Reconstr Surg, Accepted for publication.

[143] Ashjian PH, Elbarbary AS, Edmonds B, et al. In vitro differentiation of human processed lipoaspirate cells into early neural progenitors. Plast Reconstr Surg 2003;111:1922–31.

[144] Lee JA, Parrett BM, Conejero JA, et al. Biological alchemy: engineering bone and fat from fat-derived stem cells. Ann Plast Surg 2003;50:610–7.

[145] Hicok KC, Du Laney TV, Zhou YS, et al. Human adipose-derived adult stem cells produce osteoid in vivo. Tissue Eng 2004;10:371–80.

[146] Dragoo JL, Choi JY, Lieberman JR, et al. Bone induction by bmp-2 transduced stem cells derived from human fat. J Orthop Res 2003;21:622–9.

[147] Cowan CM, Shi YY, Aalami OO, et al. Adipose-derived adult stromal cells heal critical-size mouse calvarial defects. Nat Biotechnol 2004;22:560–7.

[148] Cao Y, Vacanti JP, Paige KT, et al. Transplantation of chondrocytes utilizing a polymer-cell construct to produce tissue-engineered cartilage in the shape of a human ear. Plast Reconstr Surg 1997;100:297–302.

[149] Barron V, Lyons E, Stenson-Cox C, et al. Bioreactors for cardiovascular cell and tissue growth: a review. Ann Biomed Eng 2003;31:1017–30.

[150] Fauza DO, Marler JJ, Koka R, et al. Fetal tissue engineering: diaphragmatic replacement. J Pediatr Surg 2001;36:146–51.

[151] Sodian R, Lemke T, Fritsche C, et al. Tissue-engineering bioreactors: a new combined cell-seeding and perfusion system for vascular tissue engineering. Tissue Eng 2002;8:863–70.

[152] Gabouev AI, Schultheiss D, Mertsching H, et al. In vitro construction of urinary bladder wall using porcine primary cells reseeded on acellularized bladder matrix and small intestinal submucosa. Int J Artif Organs 2003;26:935–42.

ELSEVIER
SAUNDERS

Clin Plastic Surg 32 (2005) 137–140

CLINICS IN
PLASTIC SURGERY

Index

Note: Page numbers of article titles are in **boldface** type.

A

Amastia, 74, 75

Amazia, 74

Apoptosis, cranial suture biology and, 126

Arteriovenous malformations, clinical staging of, 113
  management of, 113–114
  pathogenesis of, 112, 113

Athelia, 74, 76

B

Bionics, in treatment of brachial plexus lesions, 94

Blood vessels, malformations of, and hemangiomas,
  current management of, **99–116**
    history and physical examination in, 99–100

BMP antagonists, in cranial suture biology, 125–126

Bone replacement, current techniques for, 123

Bone tissue engineering, 128–131
  cellular therapies and, 130–131
  for complex structures, 131
  in facial trauma, 128
  scaffolds for, 129–130
  tissue regeneration in, 128–129

Botulinum injection, in obstetric brachial plexus
  palsy, 92

Brachial plexus, avulsed roots of, re-implantation of,
  in treatment of brachial plexus lesions, 93
  injury(ies) of, electrophysiologic assessment of, 83
    in infant, management of, **79–98**
    mechanism of, 80–81
    primary surgery in, 85–88
      strategies for, 88
    lesions of, nerve transfers in, 90–91
      physical therapy in, 91–92
      tendon transfers in, 90

treatment of, bionics in, 93–94
  future directions in, 93–94
  re-implantation of avulsed roots in, 93
  stem cells in, 94
repair of, primary, rationale for, 83–85
secondary deformities of, correction of, 88–90

Brachial plexus palsy, obstetric, botulinum injection
  in, 92
    epidemiology of, 79–80
    initial assessment in, 81–83
    reconstruction in, outcomes of, 92–93
    treatment of, algorithm for, 84

Breast, abnormalities of, accessory nipples, 66
  deformational, 69–71
  hyperplastic, 66–69
  hypoplastic, 71–76
  iatrogenic, 69
  pediatric, 66
  anterior thoracic hypoplasia of, 74
  bilateral absence of, 75
  burns of, 70–71, 74
  development of, 65
  giant fibroadenoma(s) of, 68, 69
  growth of, aesthetic considerations in, 65–66
  hemangioma of, 70, 72
  hyperplasia of, pediatric, 68
  hypoplasia of, following thoracostomy tube
    placement, 69, 71
  juvenile hypertrophy of, 68–69, 70
  problems of, pediatric, treatment of, **65–78**
  traumatic anomalies of, 70–71, 73
  tuberous deformity of, 72–73, 75
  tumor excision from, 70

C

Capillary-lymphaticovenous malformation, 114

Cellular therapies, and bone tissue engineering,
  130–131

Child(ren), problems of breast in. See under *Breast.*

0094-1298/05/$ – see front matter © 2005 Elsevier Inc. All rights reserved.
doi:10.1016/S0094-1298(04)00103-8

Changing Your Address?

Make sure your subscription changes too! When you notify us of your new address, you can help make our job easier by including an exact copy of your Clinics label number with your old address (see illustration below.) This number identifies you to our computer system and will speed the processing of your address change. Please be sure this label number accompanies your old address and your corrected address—you can send an old Clinics label with your number on it or just copy it exactly and send it to the address listed below.

We appreciate your help in our attempt to give you continuous coverage. Thank you.

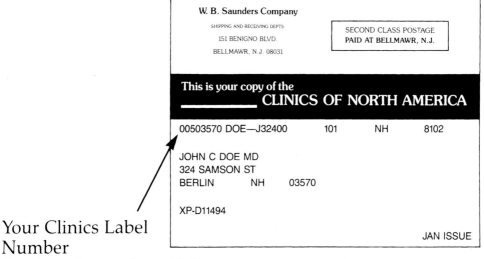

Your Clinics Label Number
Copy it exactly or send your label
along with your address to:
W.B. Saunders Company, Customer Service
Orlando, FL 32887-4800
Call Toll Free 1-800-654-2452

Please allow four to six weeks for delivery of new subscriptions and for processing address changes.